Career Readiness & Externships

Soft Skills for Pharmacy Technicians

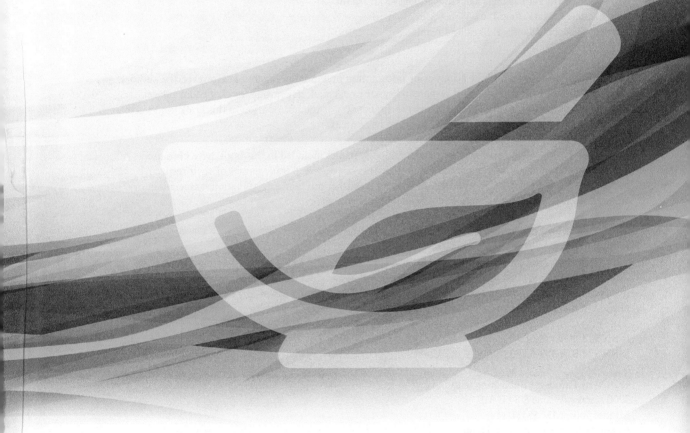

Mark Brunton, MSHE, CPhT

with Ann Cross and Martha Lanaghen

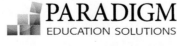

PARADIGM
EDUCATION SOLUTIONS

Minneapolis

Vice President, Content and Digital Solutions: Christine Hurney
Director of Content Development, Health Careers: Carley Fruzzetti
Developmental Editors: Carley Fruzzetti, Nancy Papsin, and Stephanie Schempp
Director of Production: Timothy W. Larson
Associate Production Editor and Project Manager: Melora Pappas
Senior Design and Production Specialist: Valerie A. King
Copy Editor: Lori Ryan
Proofreader: Shannon Kottke
Indexer: Terry Casey
Vice President, Director of Digital Products: Chuck Bratton
Digital Projects Manager: Tom Modl
Digital Solutions Manager: Gerry Yumul
Senior Director of Digital Products and Onboarding: Christopher Johnson
Supervisor of Digital Products and Onboarding: Ryan Isdahl
Vice President, Marketing: Lara Weber McLellan
Associate Product Manager: Shealan Pream

Care has been taken to verify the accuracy of information presented in this book. However, the authors, editors, and publisher cannot accept responsibility for web, email, newsgroup, or chat room subject matter or content, or for consequences from the application of the information in this book, and make no warranty, expressed or implied, with respect to its content.

Trademarks: Some of the product names and company names included in this book have been used for identification purposes only and may be trademarks or registered trade names of their respective manufacturers and sellers. The authors, editors, and publisher disclaim any affiliation, association, or connection with, or sponsorship or endorsement by, such owners.

Cover Background Illustration Credit: © iStock.com/traffic_analyzer
Interior Photo Credits: Follow the index.

We have made every effort to trace the ownership of all copyrighted material and to secure permission from copyright holders. In the event of any question arising as to the use of any material, we will be pleased to make the necessary corrections in future printings.

ISBN 978-0-76388-611-0 (print)
ISBN 978-0-76388-607-3 (digital)

© 2020 by Paradigm Publishing, LLC
7900 Xerxes Avenue S STE 310
Minneapolis, MN 55431-1118
Email: customerservice@ppij.com
Website: ParadigmEducation.com

Printed in the United States of America

27 26 25 24 23 22 21 20 19   1 2 3 4 5 6 7 8 9 10

Brief Contents

Contents

Contents

MODULE 7 Law & Ethics 133

MODULE 8   Externship Preparation & Practice   161

MODULE 9 Career Readiness, Planning, & Management 189

Preface

Career Readiness & Externships: Soft Skills for Pharmacy Technicians prepares pharmacy technician students for their externship experience and, subsequently, the workforce by providing them with soft skills training. The term *soft skills*, also known as *career-readiness skills* or *employability skills*, refers to the professional communications and behaviors, relationship skills, and personality traits that students need to achieve personal and career success. Specifically, soft skills include an individual's demonstration of:

- time management and productivity
- organizational skills
- critical thinking and problem-solving abilities
- professional appearance (hygiene practices, appropriate dress, etc.)
- professional behaviors (respect, ethics, leadership, self-direction, emotional intelligence, teamwork, work ethic, dependability, etc.)
- verbal and written professional communications
- active listening skills
- multicultural awareness and cultural competency
- career planning and management strategies

These soft skills have been recognized by business and industry leaders as being equally important to students' success in a workplace as hard skills, or the academic knowledge and technical expertise that students acquire through formal education and training programs. In fact, employers consistently cite soft skills as an area in which new employees and recent graduates need the most improvement. In a 2018 survey of 4,000 professionals, training for soft skills was identified as the top priority for talent development.[1]

In the pharmacy workplace, externship preceptors and supervisors agree that pharmacy technicians who arrive at their site for a practice experience or for entry-level employment demonstrate their academic knowledge (pharmacology,

---

[1]Dye, Lefkowitz, Pate, and Spar "2018 Workplace Learning Report," LinkedIn Learning with Lynda.com Content. https://learning.linkedin.com/content/dam/me/learning/en-us/pdfs/linkedin-learning-workplace-learning-report-2018.pdf (Accessed 10/15/19).

medical terminology, pharmacy laws and regulations, pharmacy calculations, the dispensing process, etc.). However, they are lacking the necessary soft skills to work effectively with colleagues and serve the healthcare needs of patients. For example, many students and college graduates struggle to communicate appropriately with patients, to manage their time, to think critically and solve problems, to craft a résumé, or to answer job interview questions.

Paradigm's *Career Readiness & Externships: Soft Skills for Pharmacy Technicians* addresses those needs by introducing and reinforcing the professional habits and soft skills that bridge the gap between formal education/training and externship/employment. Using examples and content specific to pharmacy technicians, this courseware provides a unique perspective on traditional soft skills and career preparation activities. Each module focuses on one of nine soft skills competencies that support the success of pharmacy technicians:

Module 1: Time Management Learn how to use time effectively and develop the time-management habits required to accomplish goals, tasks, and assignments.

Module 2: Critical Thinking & Problem Solving Learn the qualities and behaviors of critical thinkers and the methods of identifying, assessing, and navigating difficult situations.

Module 3: Professional Appearance Understand the impact of one's appearance and hygiene on professional image and career success.

Module 4: Professional Behavior Identify and exhibit professional behavior to navigate interactions and relationships with supervisors, colleagues, patients, and vendors.

Module 5: Professional Communications Develop the skills to communicate and interact skillfully and effectively with pharmacists, healthcare personnel, other pharmacy technicians, patients, and vendors.

Module 6: Multicultural Awareness & Cultural Competency Demonstrate an awareness of cultural and religious diversity and its impact on healthcare services, and ensure that colleagues and patients are treated with sensitivity and respect.

Module 7: Law & Ethics Demonstrate an understanding of pharmacy laws and regulations and exhibit ethical behavior and communications while working in a pharmacy setting.

Module 8: Externship Preparation & Practice Prepare for an externship by identifying expectations and strategies for a successful experience.

Module 9: Career Readiness, Planning, & Management Learn how to craft a résumé and cover letter, explore career options, anticipate and practice interview questions, set a career trajectory, and engage in continuing education.

Key Components

Each module offers tips, activities, and resources to support student learning. The following visual guide provides a description of these key components.

Learning Objectives address the major concepts students should learn in each module.

> ## LEARNING OBJECTIVES
>
> **1.1** Identify the seven key skills of time management.
>
> **1.2** Explain how time management is related to reliability and productivity.

Key Terms are defined both in context and in the online learning management system.

> ### Being Reliable and Productive
>
> Being **reliable** means that people can trust and depend on you. If you have a work shift, it means showing up early or on time. If you have a task to be done, it is done completely, on time, and fulfills expectations.

Think It Through scenarios challenge students to apply critical-thinking skills in their approach to addressing an issue or solving a problem.

> ### Think It Through: Planning Your Time
>
> Consider a deadline you met or a task you finished recently. Who benefited? Consider an instance in the past month when you did not complete a task as promised. Whom did your behavior affect?

Self-Reflection activities provide an opportunity for students to assess their own strengths and weaknesses and to consider strategies for improvement.

> ### Self-Reflection: What Makes You Procrastinate?
>
> *Respond to questions as honestly as possible.*
> - What tasks do you postpone or avoid?
> - How do you procrastinate? Do you check email or social media? Find other work to do? Take a break and allow yourself to get distracted? List the ways you most often fill your time when you are avoiding a task.

Expand Your Knowledge features provide additional insights into a topic covered in the module.

> ## EXPAND YOUR KNOWLEDGE
>
> **Filling a Time Jar**
> There is a popular analogy that illustrates the importance of time management by
>
> • **My "pebbles"—everyday essentials**
> These are generally recurring, ongoing

Workplace Wisdom features provide real-world examples that highlight lessons learned or advice from seasoned pharmacy professionals.

> ## WORKPLACE WISDOM
>
> **Perfecting Pharmacy Attire**
> When selecting your wardrobe to fit the dress code, choose fabrics that wear well. Cotton, while comfortable, fades and gets longer. These fabrics also are more wrinkle resistant and need less maintenance. Be sure to choose items that fit comfortably

Tables and Figures illustrate and further support the content of each module.

> **Figure 5.1 LEAD Is the Way to Handle Angry People**
>
> **L–Listen** to the customer
> **E–Explain** why it happened
> **A–Acknowledge** that it is a legitimate problem
> **D–Discuss** to decide how to resolve the issue, and thank the customer
>
>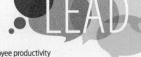
>
> Studies have demonstrated a 20% increase in employee productivity when using similar protocol to handle an angry or unsatisfied customer.

Practice Tip tips provide suggestions for best-practice approaches/techniques when working in a pharmacy.

Work Wise tips offer advice on interpersonal skills, communication, cultural awareness and sensitivity, ethical responsibility, and career preparation.

Safety Alert tips provide precautions to observe in a pharmacy.

Name Exchange tips focus on alternative names for a pharmacy or healthcare term.

Digital Assets

The modules of *Career Readiness & Externships: Soft Skills for Pharmacy Technicians* are also available within Paradigm's learning management system and provide additional resources and practice opportunities. Your instructor may assign you activities and exercises from your digital course, or you may choose to explore them on your own. The following digital resources are available to students and instructors.

Student Resources

Watch & Learn Lessons explain the concepts discussed in each module using videos, corresponding content, and a short quiz to assess your understanding of the materials.

Apply the Skills Activities provide opportunities to apply the skills taught in the module.

Critical Thinking Scenarios assess your ability to successfully navigate topic-specific scenarios.

Extension Activities provide project and exercise prompts that encourage additional investigation and insight.

Student Supplements offer additional resources and templates to accompany the module content.

Instructor Resources

Lesson Plans and other course-planning resources provide suggestions for how to best implement the *Career Readiness & Externships* product within an existing pharmacy technician program.

Answer Keys and Rubrics make it easy to assess student comprehension.

Externship Program Materials provide resources to manage externships and navigate the needs of preceptors and students. These materials include handouts and resources for students and preceptors, such as feedback templates and troubleshooting documents.

About the Authors

Mark Brunton, MSHE, CPhT

Mark Brunton has been a pharmacy technician for more than 20 years and holds a master's degree in Higher Education Administration and Leadership from Purdue University Global. He has taught, directed, and created curriculum for pharmacy technician training programs in Las Vegas for the past 12 years. Brunton's commitment to the education of pharmacy technicians stems from his passion for quality curriculum, his love of the profession, and his desire to garner respect for technicians in the field.

Brunton's experience as a preceptor made him keenly aware of the skills gap that exists between students' academic environment and the pharmacy workplace. As a result of his experience, he partnered with Paradigm Education Solutions and their JIST authors to develop a soft skills curriculum to help students and preceptors bridge that gap. He is committed to helping students attain the professional habits they need to succeed both personally and professionally.

In addition to his pharmacy technician curriculum writing, Brunton has worked as an exam-question writer for the Pharmacy Technician Certification Exam (PTCE) and served as a member of the development committee for the Certified Compounded Sterile Preparation Technician (CSPT) national certification exam overseen by the Pharmacy Technician Certification Board. Brunton is also the author of *Hospital Pharmacy Practice for Technicians* and has presented at numerous national conventions. From 2017 through 2018, Brunton served as president of the Pharmacy Technician Educators Council (PTEC). Currently, Brunton applies his skills and knowledge as the program chair for pharmacy technician education at Northwest Career College in Las Vegas.

Ann Cross and Martha Lanaghen

Ann Cross and Martha Lanaghen have worked as professionals in the career services field for more than a combined 30 years. In that time, they have consistently heard from employers across the nation that new hires possess academic knowledge and technical expertise but lack emotional intelligence and professionalism skills. For that reason, Cross and Lanaghen have implemented dozens of training programs for colleges, universities, and corporations to teach individuals desired employability skills such as professional communications and behaviors, problem solving, time management, and teamwork. According to Cross and Lanaghen, the acquisition of these skills improves individuals' ability to find a job and to keep that position.

Ann Cross has been recognized as one of the 2,000 most influential women in business for her progressive work in sales effectiveness. She has consulted with national and international companies such as Ford Motor

Company, Maytag, Sears, and General Motors. Recently, Cross was the National Director of Career Services for a large college with multiple locations. Her innovative programs led to the recognition of her college as an industry leader in student placement outcomes.

Martha Lanaghen has more than 25 years of management experience, with the vast majority of her work focused on customer and student interaction. More recently, Lanaghen was a Vice President of Student Operations at Guild Education, the acclaimed start-up organization that is changing higher education for working adults. Today, Lanaghen is a popular speaker and consultant focusing on helping online and traditional colleges build outstanding student experiences that drive student success, engagement, and, ultimately, successful employment.

Time Management

LEARNING OBJECTIVES

1 Identify the seven key skills of time management. (Section 1.1)

2 Explain how time management is related to reliability and productivity. (Section 1.1)

3 Implement strategies for practicing good time management. (Section 1.1)

4 Create manageable monthly, weekly, and daily to-do lists. (Section 1.2)

5 Describe tactics to prevent multitasking, interruptions, and distractions. (Section 1.3)

6 Understand the challenges associated with procrastination and how to overcome them. (Section 1.3)

7 Apply punctuality strategies. (Section 1.4)

8 Explain the importance of and strategies to organizing your workspace. (Section 1.5)

To view the *ASHP/ACPE Accreditation Standards* addressed in this chapter, refer to Appendix A.

Have you ever forgotten an appointment or been late for class? Have you ever spent too much time on one task, so you couldn't get something else done? Imagine not being able to finish filling prescriptions or IV preparations in the allotted time frame because you were distracted on the job.

As you work to meet your educational and professional goals, you need to manage your time effectively. This module walks you through the steps necessary to effectively manage your time. Some of the topics addressed include setting a time budget, creating to-do lists, preventing distractions and procrastination, being punctual, and organizing your workspace.

1.1 Time Management

Time management helps you complete goals and tasks by their deadlines without constant supervision or reminders. Wikipedia defines **time management** as, "the process of planning and exercising conscious control of time spent on specific activities, especially to increase effectiveness, efficiency, or productivity." Time management involves different skills, tools, and strategies that people apply in various ways depending on their personalities and lifestyles.

Time-management skills and methodologies can work at both the macro and micro level. For example, effective time management skills can help you accomplish weekly, monthly, or even annual tasks. These skills can also be used on a minute-to-minute or hourly basis to complete daily school or work objectives.

By learning and practicing macro time-management skills now, as a pharmacy technician student, you can then apply these skills at the micro level when dealing with patients when you start your career as a pharmacy technician.

Controlling your time requires several different skills, including:

- sorting and prioritizing tasks
- estimating the amount of time per task
- scheduling your tasks and deadlines
- making your daily to-do list
- preventing multitasking, interruptions, distractions, and procrastination
- putting an emphasis on being punctual
- organizing your workspace to maximize efficiency

These interrelated skills can become habits through repeated practice. Some of these skills will come easier than others, but all of them can be learned. These skills are necessary in any pharmacy position you take, because your daily work will often go at a fast pace. With calls on hold and customers waiting, or nursing floors needing to be restocked, good time management will be one of your most useful assets. You will need these skills so that employers, coworkers, customers, and patients find you reliable and productive.

Think It Through: Planning Your Time

Consider a deadline you met or a task you finished recently. Who benefited? Consider an instance in the past month when you did not complete a task as promised. Whom did your behavior affect?

Being Reliable and Productive

Being **reliable** means that people can trust and depend on you. If you have a work shift, it means showing up early or on time. If you have a task to be done, it is done completely, on time, and fulfills expectations.

Being **productive** means using your time efficiently to get more done. If you work in a community pharmacy, you may have duties for dispensing, keeping your work space clean, or checking expiration dates on medications. Your priority as a pharmacy technician will be serving patients and dispensing their medications. You can work on the other tasks when there are no patients waiting. Using the time in between patients in this way allows you to be productive. Pharmacists are looking for reliability and productivity in the pharmacy technicians they hire.

You are likely to find that time management skills are applicable not only for professional goals and assignments but for personal ones as well. You may also see your energy and mood elevate as you intentionally choose how you spend your days.

Considering Your Current Time-Management Habits

Time is a resource you spend, like money. The difference is that everyone has the exact same amount of time each day. Because you can't increase the number of hours in a day, you must make the most of those hours and minutes. This skill requires building a detailed awareness of how you currently spend your time and making choices about how you want to spend your time going forward.

> "Time is a resource you spend, like money."

Self-Reflection:
How Well Do You Manage Your Time?

Evaluate your level of skill in each of the areas below, from 1 to 5, with 1 being the lowest and 5 being the highest ranking. Respond to statements as honestly as possible.

Questions	1	2	3	4	5
How well do you think you use your time?					
How consistent are you in meeting personal goal deadlines?					

Continues...

Questions	1	2	3	4	5
How consistent are you in meeting deadlines assigned by others?					
How happy are you with the amount of work you produce?					
How happy are you with the amount of work you produce?					
How organized and productive are you with your projects?					
How organized are your workspace, tools, and files?					
How efficient do you think you are in fulfilling tasks?					
How efficient do you think others feel you are?					
How well do you stay focused and avoid distractions?					
How well do you feel others would say you follow through on tasks?					
How well do you allot time for and clean up after the tasks are complete?					

Tally Your Score: _____ x 1 = _____ ; _____ x 2 = _____ ; _____ x 3 = _____ ; _____ x 4 = _____ ; _____ x 5 = _____

Total Score: _____

46 to 60 points: This score indicates you have a very strong foundation for time management.

26 to 45 points: This score indicates that you are familiar with time management and may have some success achieving goals. You can practice the skills to achieve more.

Below 26 points: This score indicates a need for immediate attention. You are not currently managing your time well. It is recommended that you establish a plan to begin using time-management techniques, and work to implement them in all tasks.

Prioritizing How You Spend Your Time

The order you do tasks matters. You will be able to fit more important elements into your life and get more of your everyday duties done if you prioritize the most important tasks ahead of recreation or optional tasks.

To **prioritize** means to sort by level of importance. The first step in time management will be to sort the major tasks and actions of your life into the different piles by level of importance. Then prioritize the elements within each category. Ask yourself: How many important things can be done in one day? How much time can be devoted to each task?

You must do similar decision making for everyday essentials—which ones are the most important per day? Per week? Per month?

By thinking about how you currently fill your days versus how you would ideally like to, you can be more thoughtful and strategic about your choices. Making conscious choices about how you fill your time may also help you live at a less hectic pace, with more rest in between tasks.

Filling a Time Jar

There is a popular analogy that illustrates the importance of time management by comparing the hours in a day to a jar, which we fill with different elements. Everyone has the same size jar, but we all fill it up differently. How we prioritize our tasks and fill our time determines whether we can complete all the tasks planned for a single day. Watch the time jar analogy for effective time management: **https://SSPharm .ParadigmEducation.com/TimeJar.**

The elements that we put in our time jars are:

- **My "rocks"—important tasks**
  These are the responsibilities and tasks that must be done to meet your goals or to fulfill obligations to family members or friends. These tasks often have existing scheduled times (e.g., class times, lab times, job schedule, childcare, family events).

- **My "pebbles"—everyday essentials**
  These are generally recurring, ongoing tasks that must be done to keep your life going (e.g., making meals, doing household chores, paying bills, personal hygiene, sleeping).

- **My "sand"—recreation**
  These are generally tasks that you do for fun (e.g., looking at social media, hanging out with friends, playing video games, watching movies, engaging in a hobby).

The key to this analogy is figuring out how important various elements of your life are and what order you put the items into the jar. What happens if you put in the sand, then the pebbles, then the rocks? Can you get the same amounts of the important rocks into the jar? What happens when you reverse the order? Experiment on your own or in class by inserting the rocks, pebbles, and sand in different orders into the jar.

1.2 Time-Management Skills and Strategies

Now that you have considered the way you fill your time, you can probably see areas in which you can use your time more effectively. To do so, it helps to have tools, strategies, and skills. The following are common time-management techniques:

- Gather time planning tools.
- Make lists of tasks.
- Prioritize tasks for the month, week, and day.
- Create a time budget.
- Manage tasks in a calendar.
- Make to-do lists for the day.

Each of these skills requires some explanation and practice, but are important to effectively managing your time.

Gathering Time-Planning Tools

Before you begin, you'll need the right tools—a notepad or notepad app along with a daily calendar, personal planner, or scheduling app. These tools allow you to make lists and take note of any scheduled dates for classes, work, meetings, gatherings, and other events that are important to you in one or two organized places. Do not rely solely on your memory.

A calendar/planner and its segmented blocks are the bones in the body of your time plan. They give you the structure that you need to plan your tasks. It is difficult to manage your time if you can't see your appointments or due dates in the context of a date, week, month, and year.

Writing Out Monthly and Weekly Lists

To manage your time, it's essential to write down the important tasks you need to complete in the week and month ahead to meet your long-term and short-term goals. You also need to add to the lists the necessary tasks for living and meeting your family, school, and work responsibilities.

Experts find that the list-making step accomplishes many things, such as allowing you to not worry as much, to be more accountable, prioritize better, to delegate, create realistic expectations, and affirm your progress.

Reduces Worrying Most people carry around worries about the things they need to do that they might forget. When you write down a task, you remove the worry about forgetting it.

Improves Your Accountability When your list is shared with others, it gives you a tool to hold yourself accountable. This is like posting a before picture to social media prior to starting a workout program. Engaging with others can motivate you to keep on task.

Allows You to Prioritize A list allows you to create order out of the chaos of unrelated thoughts and tasks. Once you write things down, you have the power to consider their necessity and move them around in order of importance. This will be discussed in greater detail in the next section.

Allows You to Cancel or Delegate Items Looking at a list, you can decide if you can delegate some tasks to others. You can also delete or postpone unimportant or distracting items. Learning when to delete items is as important as adding them.

Allows You to Make Realistic Expectations If you find that you have too many major items on your daily or weekly list, you may need to reconsider your expectations. Are you setting yourself up for failure? Have you committed yourself to too many things?

Affirms Your Progress One of the greatest things about to-do lists is the act of completing items. You achieve a sense of satisfaction and accomplishment when viewing everything that you have already accomplished as you go down the list.

Prioritizing the Tasks on Your Lists

A long list can feel overwhelming, however, not every item on the list is equally important. One of the hardest things to learn is how to say "no" or "not right now." You can move some items to a later time. Since we all have many options for how to spend our time each day, prioritization is key.

Once you have listed what you need to get done, it's time to prioritize. Sort each task into one of four categories—urgent (U), important (I), necessary (N), or marginal (M).

Urgent work—U This is work that must be accomplished immediately. For example, if you are working to achieve a passing grade for a pharmacology course, you must consider many factors. While reading all the required chapters for the term is essential, it may not be urgent. There might be a drug terms quiz tomorrow and that you should study for first, and therefore takes priority.

Important work—I These are tasks which must be completed to get the job done, but don't have an immediate deadline associated with them. In the pharmacy, putting away the daily order of medications must get done and has a deadline, but it doesn't have to happen immediately for work to continue. Therefore, this task is important, but it doesn't necessarily have to happen first thing.

Necessary work—N This work is important but not tied to any other task, nor is it work that must happen right away. In the pharmacy example, checking expiration dates of medications on the shelf is important, but it can be done with some flexibility, and if it doesn't get done that day, all other work can continue as needed.

Marginal work—M This work consists of tasks that are less important or do not have an assigned deadline, but you would like to get them done when you can. For example, dusting the medication shelves shows attention to detail, but if it did not happen on a regular basis, it would not be immediately noticed. Be aware that marginal work, if left for too long, can rise in priority, (e.g., undusted shelves will become noticeable later, if given enough time).

Determine the Category To determine a task's priority level, ask yourself, what will happen if I don't get this done? What are the consequences? The level and timing of the consequences determines whether the task is urgent, important, necessary, or marginal. This prioritization process is based on the individual. It depends on how you value different tasks and their outcomes.

Practice Tip

It's common to consider all your tasks urgent. This makes prioritizing your work nearly impossible. Compare tasks to each other for overall perspective.

Table 1.1 shows how this works for different tasks on a list. Joshua listed his goals at a weekly, monthly, and yearly level with their priority level.

Table 1.1 Sample of Joshua's Tasks Lists		
Week's Tasks	**Month's Tasks**	**Year's Major Tasks**
Study for end-of-chapter test—I	Pass current course—U	Complete finals (May)—I
Go grocery shopping—N	Pay bills—I	Look for new apartment—N
Spend time with significant other—N	Spend time with Jose and Letitia—M	Have a Fourth of July barbecue—M
Work out—M	Increase running time and distance—M	Run an obstacle race—M
Complete homework assignments—I	Go to anniversary dinner—N	Complete externship—I
Declutter apartment—M	Practice interviewing—N	Study for certification exam (June)—I
Fix chair—N	Ask mentor about externship—N	Take certification exam (July)—I
Call phone company—N	Get bus pass—N	Start applying for jobs (August)—I
Visit Uncle Jedidiah—I	Clean bathroom—N	Buy a new/used car—I

 WORKPLACE WISDOM

Pharmacy Prioritization

In a community pharmacy dispensing position, you will likely have to prioritize your tasks on an ongoing basis, and priorities will shift depending on context. Should you ask a customer at the window to wait while you are completing a prescription fill, or should you stop the dispensing process and help the customer? Then the phone rings. Do you answer it or continue in one of these tasks? When do you ask for help and from whom?

Your orientation and policies and procedure manual should provide you with guidelines on how to prioritize. The exact amount of time each interruption will take may also make a difference in how you prioritize.

The nature of a task will also help you decide what to do. If you are in the middle of calculations or something critical to safety, its priority is higher and must be completed before helping the customer. If, however, you are just preparing to fill a prescription and a customer appears to be in a hurry, the priority might be to help the customer first and then return to filling the prescription.

Learning to prioritize tasks in your academic career will help you quickly prioritize tasks when you are on the job.

Building a Time Budget

Once you have figured out your priorities and deadlines, consider how much time each task might take. This is a list where you set aside, or budget, the time needed to do the task well. A **budget** is a plan that estimates and allots resources (such as time or money) based on listed categories and their priorities. Using your time budget, you will be better able to schedule tasks out on a calendar or in a planner because you are setting aside enough time to get them done.

The first step in budgeting your time is estimating how long each of your tasks will take. In some cases, such as "attending lab class," you'll know how long the task takes based on its specific time limit and your experience. In other situations, you'll need to estimate the length of time needed, such as travel time to and from said lab. Afterward, you'll have to check how accurate your estimate was for future planning.

With your estimate and task lists, you can build a weekly budget (as illustrated in Table 1.2), and from this, a daily budget.

Table 1.2 Allana's Weekly Time Budget

Activity	Deadline	Rank	Time Needed	When I Will Do This
Pharmacy lecture classes plus moving between classes	End of semester	I	5 hours/day	M, W, F
Pharmacy lab classes plus moving between classes	End of semester	I	5 hours/day	T, Th
Study for tests/ assignments	Tests T, Th, F; projects M, W Sat general	I	2 hours/day	M, T, W, Th 2 hours (2 hours night), Sat 2 hours
Work	N/A	I	11 hours/week	F, Sat
Wash laundry	Need work clothes by F	N	1 hours/week	W after dinner before second study time
Work out	N/A	N	4 hours/week	T, Th, 6 a.m. Sun afternoon or evening
Explore and apply for externships	End of semester	N	2 hours	Sun
Pay bills	Do by F, rent due	U	1 hour	?
Fix tire on bike	By Sun for bike ride	N	1 hour	?
Call Mom	End of week	N	½ hour	?
Meet with Charlie	End of month	N	2 hours	?
Watch favorite shows	N/A	M		?

Managing Your Calendar

Figuring out your task list, prioritizing tasks with deadlines, estimating the amount of time needed for each task, and building your time budget may seem like many steps to complete. But as you practice time-management skills, you will be able to do them more automatically and naturally. You will find methods that fit you best and may be doing many of these tasks already.

The next step is to use your time budget to schedule your tasks in a planner or calendar. An example of a weekly calendar is illustrated in Table 1.3. Maintaining a schedule will help keep you focused and organized. You'll be able to track your progress, and not worry about whether you will forget an appointment or deadline. Saying no to distractions and diversions that come along will be easier, because you can see that you have something already scheduled.

Table 1.3 Allana's Weekly Planner							
Time	**Mon**	**Tue**	**Wed**	**Thu**	**Fri**	**Sat**	**Sun**
6:00 AM		Go to gym		Go to gym			
7:00 AM							
8:00 AM						Work	
9:00 AM	Lecture Class	Lab Class	Lecture Class	Lab Class	Lecture Class	Work	
10:00 AM	Lecture Class	Lab Class	Lecture Class	Lab Class	Lecture Class	Work	
11:00 AM	Lecture Class	Lab Class	Lecture Class	Lab Class	Lecture Class	Work	
12:00 PM	Lecture Class	Lab Class	Lecture Class	Lab Class	Lecture Class	Work	
1:00 PM	Lecture Class	Lab Class	Lecture Class	Lab Class	Lecture Class	Work	
2:00 PM	Lecture Class	Lab Class	Lecture Class	Lab Class	Lecture Class	Work	Go to gym
3:00 PM						Work	Go to gym
4:00 PM							Externship Search
5:00 PM	Project Study	Test Study	Project Study	Test Study	Test Study	General Study	

Continues…

Career Readiness & Externships: Soft Skills for Pharmacy Technicians

Allana's Weekly Planner ...*continued*

Time	Mon	Tue	Wed	Thu	Fri	Sat	Sun
6:00 PM	Project Study	Test Study	Project Study	Test Study	Test Study	General Study	
7:00 PM							
8:00 PM			Laundry		Work	Meet w/ Charlie	
9:00 PM					Work	Meet w/ Charlie	
10:00 PM					Work		

The following are tips to schedule deadlines, consider others, schedule tasks at logical times, minimize distractions, practice accountability, and celebrate progress, all which will help you successfully manage your calendar.

Schedule Deadlines Schedule all the deadlines you know first. This ensures the essentials are in place first. Another strategy is to mark deadlines down for an earlier time. By doing this, you add buffer time. If you are working on a big project, give yourself an extra day or week in advance of the deadline. If it is a small project, give yourself a few extra hours. This gives you time to double-check your work. It allows time for surprises and unexpected emergencies. Getting your work done early builds trust with your colleagues and supervisors.

Make sure to add in transition and buffer time. When you are scheduling tasks in your planner, don't schedule things too tightly on any one day. Schedule time between tasks for breaks and travel time. You need down time and flexibility for surprises. If someone suddenly needs you for something important or your computer stops working, you must be able to adapt and rearrange your schedule to accommodate the situation. Also, you may find you have been too optimistic about how quickly you work and have not scheduled enough time to properly complete a project.

Assign your own due dates/times for tasks without deadlines. Base your due date on how long the tasks take and when you'd ideally like them done.

Consider Others Take special note of the tasks for which others depend upon you to get done. Be very careful to schedule deadlines in advance of when others are waiting for you. This thoughtfulness builds trust.

Add extra time when your work depends on others. For instance, you cannot finish your externship application until you have gotten letters of recommendation. Make sure you ask instructors, employers, and friends who will be writing your letters as soon as you know you need them to allow for sufficient writing time. Then give the letter writers a due date a little in advance of the application deadline. Schedule the task into your calendar to check in and follow up periodically.

Schedule Tasks at Logical Times Schedule tasks at the right time of day, if possible. For instance, if you have creative work, do it when you are most creative and have the fewest distractions. For morning people, this will likely be before others wake up. For night people, it is often after others have gone to bed. Develop the habit of thinking about the appropriateness of timing for certain tasks.

Consider grouping similar activities together. Highly productive people know that you lose valuable time when you start and stop tasks, so they schedule similar tasks together. If you must go to the computer lab for two different classes, you can combine those study times together. If you have several meals to prepare in a week, you can do them all on one day and heat them up on the assigned day.

Another strategy is to schedule certain days for routine weekly tasks. In the 1900s, many American homemakers used specific days of the week for certain chores (e.g., Monday, washing; Tuesday, ironing; Wednesday, mending; Thursday, shopping; Friday, baking; Saturday, cleaning: Sunday, day of rest). This was a way to divide and prioritize ongoing essential tasks over a full week, rather than all at once. The strategy is sound for many other tasks as well. For instance, some people still do chores on Saturday morning, have family time on Sunday, and use certain early mornings for exercise or laundry.

Minimize Interruptions There is a reason that quiet libraries have been recommended for study for centuries. It is easier to concentrate and be productive when you are not being presented with the options of conversation, TV, movies, video games, or other tasks that need to be done. Scheduling times during your day to go to a room with few distractions to get difficult tasks done is more effective.

Practice Accountability People are social creatures, and they tend to do better when they can do things with a friend or task partner who is dedicated to the same goal. Physical tasks, such as exercise, are more fun when done with others. Studying for a test can also be productive with partners or study groups. Teaming up with others who can quality check your work can be a very useful and productive technique to get more done with better results.

Remember that reading aloud, getting others' feedback, proofreading, clean-up, and follow-through on projects and tasks take time. Schedule in time for quality checks and clean-up.

Celebrate Progress Make sure you schedule in mini celebrations for the times when you meet some of your short-term goals. Reward yourself in some way, perhaps with a coffee, happy hour, or meal when you have reached a goal.

Making and Using Your Daily To-Do List

With your weekly schedule filled in with required tasks, it is time to make a to-do list for the day. This is going from the macro to the micro level of time management. The following are time-saving productivity techniques and cautions to use when making your to-do list and scheduling the tasks in your daily planner.

Be Realistic Don't overwhelm yourself with a list that's too long. The point of the list is to make you feel productive when items are completed. If the list is too intimidating due to its length, it will have the opposite effect.

Attack the Most Important and Hardest Tasks First Mark Twain said, "If it's your job to eat a frog, it's best to do it first thing in the morning. And if it's your job to eat two frogs, it's best to eat the biggest one first." The biggest and hardest task should be done first in your day, when your energy is highest.

Do Quick Things Between Harder Tasks Every list should also have a few simple and swift tasks sprinkled in so that you can complete these in between other things and check them off. This gives you momentum in your productivity.

Combine Tasks Sometimes physical tasks have wait times built in that you can use for a different task. For instance, if you have a long commute, you could use the time stuck in traffic to listen to a podcast about pharmacy. Or you may

WORKPLACE WISDOM

Pomo-what?

When I was working to earn my bachelor's degree online, I had a full-time job as a program director as well as a part-time weekend job, with very little time left over. I know these challenges were like what many of my students faced, and I truly understood how hard it could be to study, complete assignments, have a life, and still find time to even sleep!

It was hard to concentrate and stay focused, with my attention wandering and my grades slipping. I researched productivity "hacks" and found an article on the Pomodoro technique. The Pomodoro technique consists of 20 minutes of intense concentration and then a 10-minute rest. This method was developed by Francesco Cirillo,

an entrepreneur and author who developed the method as a university student trying to get his studies done efficiently.

There was a link to an online timer as well as a phone app with an alarm set to keep users on the 20/10-minute schedule.

It felt very much like a high-intensity workout, with quick bursts of energy and short recovery times. When I tried it for studying and working on papers, I found I was able to accomplish more in a shorter period, increasing my productivity.

I have used it since to get my master's degree as well as write my first book—all while keeping my sanity somewhat intact.

—Mark Brunton, MSHE, CPhT

need to exercise but also need to get to class, biking to school can solve both of these objectives.

Remember Small Ongoing Tasks Don't delay marginal or less necessary work too long. Maintenance work and other work that might seem less urgent can be put off so long that it may rise in level of importance. For instance, it can be a problem if you delay cleaning or organizing your files or workspace because when you need to find an item, your space will be too cluttered. Schedule maintenance and clean-up tasks on a regular basis.

Work Using Intervals You can build up concentration and productivity by practicing incremental breaks from any task. The brain works like a muscle, and you can improve its capabilities and focus with practice. While reading and working on tasks that require focus and thought, work to build up your concentration. For instance, read a paragraph or two and then look up to consider what you just read. Then read a few more paragraphs before looking up to think again. Continue this pattern, and you will find that over time, you will gradually build up your reading and focus skills. This method is also used in physical training, known as High Intensity Interval Training (HIIT), or the Pomodoro technique, for large task completion.

Include Time Outdoors Spend time outdoors each day, whether biking to work, taking the dog for a walk, or exercising. Too much time with electronics can reduce your ability to concentrate, but nature can have the opposite effect. Scientists have found that even looking outside to a scene with trees while studying or working can improve your outcomes. Time outdoors can do even more to improve your focus, memory, mood, creativity, energy, and productivity while reducing stress.

1.3 Common Enemies of Time Management

There are many reasons that time-management strategies can fail. The most common is a failure to stick to it consistently. Other challenges include multitasking, interruptions, recreation and screen time distractions, and procrastination.

Avoiding Multitasking

Many people think multitasking is a beneficial skill, and something to aspire to. Psychological studies, however, have found that multitasking is a myth. Your mind cannot focus on two things at once so it switches back and forth, losing focus each time as it must remember or reorient itself to each task. This greatly reduces productivity, causing tasks to take longer than they would have if you had focused on one task at a time.

EXPAND YOUR KNOWLEDGE

Dangers of Whistling While You Work

Whistling while you work is great for chores around your home. But singing or listening to music with lyrics while studying, dispensing medication, or performing other tasks that require concentration can be self-defeating and even dangerous.

Science has shown that the brain will often focus on the sound of the voice and any lyrics. It is like trying to speak to someone on the phone while watching television. However, music or sounds of nature without words does not draw conscious focus. That is why classical music can

enhance concentration. If that is not your favorite genre, there are productivity playlists that have popular music with the lyrics removed for the same purpose. Here are some articles to consider:

- "Does Music Really Help You Concentrate?" by Dean Burnett. https://SSPharm.ParadigmEducation.com/Music
- "Top 5 Reasons to Listen to Classical Music While Studying" by CMUSE. https://SSPharm.ParadigmEducation.com/ClassicalMusic

Multitasking also raises the risk of making greater errors, which is problematic in pharmacy. In fact, this is commonly referred to as a **capture error**, in which the technician's attention is captured by something else while dispensing, such as answering a phone while entering a prescription. It's difficult to avoid multitasking, but, awareness of the risks can help.

Eliminate the Urge to Multitask The following are some techniques and tips to use to avoid the habit of multitasking. Some of these tips are made up of the other elements of time management discussed in this module.

Use Apps There are many applications and websites you can use to limit your access to distracting content while working. These can be set to block website time wasters for a specific amount of time and can allow you to specify which sites and applications to block.

Mute or Disable Notifications The icons that tell us new content is available grab our attention and distract us from tasks at hand. Turning them off or muting for a time can allow more focus on directed activities.

Clean Your Workspace A cluttered desk or work area can draw your focus from one activity to another. Less mess equals less distraction. Organizing your workspace will be discussed in greater detail later in this module.

Reducing Interruptions

Being interrupted can reduce efficiency and your ability to stick to your time-management planning. Pharmacy technicians get very little uninterrupted time to work on their high-priority tasks. They must deal with phone calls, information requests, and a whole host of other events that crop up unexpectedly. Some events need to be dealt with immediately, but others can wait to be managed. To successfully manage interruptions in the pharmacy, you will want to consider various interruption-reduction strategies to best address big interruptions that you have control over.

One way to manage interruptions is by alerting others that you are unavailable for a period. For work, this could mean asking the customer on the phone to hold while you complete a task. At home, this could include closing your door (if possible) or placing a sign outside your workspace. These simple actions let others know that you don't want to be interrupted.

Another way to manage interruptions is to let your calls go to voice mail and set up an automatic response for texts or emails. You can simply write, "Your message is important to me. I will be unavailable to answer emails or take calls from 9:00 to 11:00 a.m. today; however, I will respond this afternoon when available. If the matter is urgent, please contact _____." This automatic reply will help senders know that their messages aren't being ignored and allows them to go about their own business with a reasonable expectation of when you will respond.

> ### Think It Through: Handling Interruptions
> What interruptions do you usually encounter during your day, and how do you handle them? How will you adapt your current strategies for handling interruptions for your future job as a pharmacy technician?

Triumphing Over Major Distractions

In addition to the problems of multitasking and physical interruptions, there are mental distractions, such as recreation time, screen time, time spent worrying, repeating work, and hoarding information.

Analyze Your Recreational Time Choices Recreational time often goes by without being noticed. In moderation, recreation is healthy and useful. If you are not careful, however, recreation can turn into a source of great distraction. For instance, playing in a local community basketball team has the benefits of health and wellness and stress relief. But going to a bar with friends and staying out later than you intended will make it hard to go to class or work the next morning.

Understand the Dangers of Screen Time Most of us spend significant amounts of time a day looking at screens without noticing it. We check our smartphones and computers for texts, emails, and Snapchat, Instagram, and Facebook notifications. Studies show that when a notification alert sounds, our minds react by emitting dopamine, a pleasure hormone in our brains.

EXPAND YOUR KNOWLEDGE

Screen Time—the Unnoticed Time Sap

In 2016, a Nielsen Company report found that the average American spends more than half the waking hours of a day staring at a screen. The average time on media was 10 hours and 39 minutes in 2016, an hour more than was reported in 2015.

The 10 hours adds up to 74.5 waking hours per week—almost 3 full days of the week! That may be why many people say they don't have enough time for studying, fitness, volunteering, and other goals. For more information on the Nielsen report, see "Americans Devote More than 10 Hours a Day to Screen Time, and Growing" by Jacqueline Howard. https://SSPharm.ParadigmEducation.com/ScreenTime

Video games provide similar responses. The World Health Organization calls an overuse of gaming a condition called *gaming disorder*, because the flashing images and action can be so addictive.

When using screens, time often flies by without thought. We can lose hours per day without realizing it, and then we get stressed when we don't accomplish our goals or complete our job assignments.

Finally, another concern when spending too much time on smartphones and computers is that it can reduce our time interacting directly with other people. Studies have found that overuse of social media can decrease our ability to interact with others in face-to-face situations effectively.

For all these reasons, psychologists and time-management specialists recommend that individuals consciously limit their screen time and schedule daily breaks physically away from phones, computers, TVs, and videos games.

Avoid Common Time Wasters When you understand the factors that are working against you, staying on task becomes much easier. Some common time wasters include worrying too much, repeating work, and hoarding unnecessary information.

Worrying Trying to predict the future can take up a lot of our time. Keeping a journal, discussing worries with friends and family, or even meditation can all help to alleviate worries.

Repeating Work Rereading the same information more than once, not taking good notes and having to go back for clarification, or not saving your work (and then losing the data) are all examples of work that ends up needing to be redone. Focusing your attention can eliminate the need to reread items, using advanced note taking skills (e.g., Cornell Method, Split Page, etc.), and autosaving applications are all ways to overcome this pitfall.

Hoarding Unnecessary Information This time killer is mostly related to email and junk mail, but clutter and information overload are also time wasters. There are many strategies on the web for how to manage email inboxes as well as your desktop. Find a strategy that works for you and stick to it.

Preventing Procrastination

Most problems you encounter while trying to stick to your time-management lists and schedules are external. Procrastination, however, is an internal challenge. **Procrastination** is the act of delaying or postponing a task.

Have you ever put off completing something difficult or uninteresting? People often avoid challenging projects due to a fear of failure, or they avoid projects that seem boring, annoying, or frustrating, even if they are necessary.

Procrastination wastes valuable time. Routine tasks that could have been done sooner become more urgent and sometimes more complicated the closer they are to the deadline. In addition, if you procrastinate, you are very likely to make avoidable mistakes as you rush to finish.

As with all the other time-management skills, there are tips and tricks you can use. Doing a little bit at a time, conquering your fears, putting tasks into the larger context, and delegating can all help you prevent or overcome procrastination.

Break Up Large Tasks An old African proverb states: How do you eat an elephant? One bite at a time. Cut big tasks you are likely to put off into small ones. Then celebrate each small task completed as a victory.

> "Always do what you are most afraid to do."

Conquer Your Fears Ralph Waldo Emerson said about work, "Always do what you are most afraid to do." Emerson was talking about our inner fears of failure, of trying things when we are not yet confident. Take the risk to leap bravely into the work that is the hardest. It is likely to contain the most potential for growth and accomplishment.

See the Bigger Picture For the tasks that seem tedious, boring, or unimportant, try looking at them in a different light. They are unappealing unless you can see them in the larger context of what they help accomplish. They are necessary for a reason, and that reason can provide meaning and motivation for the individual tasks. For example, restocking medication vials is often seen as very tedious and boring, but in the larger context, having them available at the peak of production enables you to complete prescription fills quickly and efficiently.

Delegate or Reduce Responsibilities Procrastination often happens when people become overwhelmed. You may have too much work or see so much to do that you don't know where to begin. See if there are some tasks you can ask someone else can do or consider if you have taken on too many responsibilities. Maybe you will need to shed some commitments to focus on your most important goals and values.

Self-Reflection: What Makes You Procrastinate?

Respond to questions as honestly as possible.

- What tasks do you postpone or avoid?
- How do you procrastinate? Do you check email or social media? Find other work to do? Take a break and allow yourself to get distracted? List the ways you most often fill your time when you are avoiding a task.
- How does your procrastination affect your work?

1.4 Punctuality

One of the key components of reliability is punctuality. **Punctuality** means consistently arriving where you are supposed to be when you are supposed to be there. Punctuality allows supervisors, coworkers, family members, and friends to depend on you.

When employees are punctual, the workplace operates more smoothly as a whole. Remember that there are coworkers either waiting to end their shifts or start the day who rely on you to be on time.

If you don't show up on time and many customers come into the pharmacy at once, dispensing can get very backed up. Customers may get frustrated and not return to the pharmacy. This harms the business overall, and you may get reprimanded or even terminated. In many states, there are regulations dictating how many technicians and pharmacists can be on duty during a shift. These are known as pharmacist-to-technician ratios. If a pharmacist is late, several technicians cannot begin work until the pharmacist arrives. A pharmacy is a team where everyone depends upon each other. If anyone is late, there can be repercussions for the rest of the workday as everyone struggles to catch up with their work.

Understanding the Importance of Punctuality

Punctuality flows from good time management. In a 2016 CareerBuilder survey, more than 4 in 10 employers reported having fired workers for being late. Employers are also less likely to promote employees who are chronically late. The CareerBuilder survey reported that 16 percent of American workers were late once per week.

Do you fall into this statistic? Chronic excuses for being late, such as over-sleeping, procrastinating, and traffic, are not acceptable to employers. These can be eliminated with better time management and organization.

Some cultures have a less rigid view of punctuality. This approach can be acceptable outside of working hours, but in most American workplaces (especially those that are highly scheduled), this is not acceptable. Pharmacies are usually tightly scheduled. Technicians need to adapt to the work culture and expectations of the pharmacy to function there well. It is essential to arrive at work when your employer and coworkers expect you to.

Self-Reflection:
The Effects of Being Early and Late

Complete the following self-assessment. Respond as honestly as possible.
Consider a recent event when you arrived early. How did you feel? What were the effects on others? What were the consequences for you?

Consider an event where you arrived late. How did you feel? What were the effects on others? What were the consequences for you?

Practicing Punctuality Techniques

Punctuality is easier to consistently achieve when you have strategies. Even if you are someone who tends to be late, you can train yourself to be on time by first examining how long getting ready really takes, making sure to account for weather and traffic, and avoiding last-minute distractions. Other tips include scheduling yourself a 10 to 15-minute buffer time, setting alarms, and alerting people if you cannot avoid being late.

Examine How Long Getting Ready Takes Many people who are chronically late are overly optimistic and considerably underestimate how much time it takes to shower, dress, eat breakfast, etc. Always allow for extra time.

Check Weather and Traffic Conditions To avoid delays, check the status of traffic and weather an hour before leaving in case you need to make plans for alternative routes or methods to arrive on time.

Avoid Last-Minute Distractions People often get distracted from arriving on time by doing something they think will take only a minute, but then it takes a lot longer, such as answering a phone call, checking Facebook, or answering an email.

Schedule Yourself 10 to 15 Minutes Early Like giving yourself due dates ahead of your final deadline as a buffer, you need to do the same for all appointments. Plan to be there 15 minutes ahead of time, and you will usually end up on time even if there are unexpected delays.

Set Incremental Alarms People need time for their minds to adjust to going from one place to another. Just like a wake-up alarm with the snooze button or parents who give their kids 10- and 5-minute warnings about leaving soon, use reminders to stay conscious of time. Some people even set their clocks 5 or 10 minutes ahead to force themselves to get going early.

Alert Someone if You Must Be Late If you must be late because of an unavoidable difficulty, call or text ahead to let those waiting know, so they don't worry. Let them know when you will arrive and what to do in the meantime.

1.5 The Importance of an Organized Space

Organizing your space will boost your time efficiency, reliability, productivity, and punctuality. Consider that if you are constantly looking for the right file, measurement instrument, your keys, your wallet, or your glasses, you will waste a lot of time. Progress is delayed on all other tasks until the needed items are found. Being disorganized can affect your work performance.

In the pharmacy, being disorganized can also severely affect safety and team efficiency. When clutter invades the pharmacy, it can influence others' performance.

If things in your workspace and your life are sorted into the most appropriate places, you will easily find them when you need them. You will also feel more in control and less stressed.

 Self-Reflection:
Check How Organized You Are

For each of the statements, mark the appropriate box to rate your habit: "always," "sometimes," or "rarely/never." Respond to statements as honestly as possible.

Statement	Always	Sometimes	Rarely/Never
I have a designated place for all my things at work.			
I have a designated place for all my things at home.			
I have a regular routine for putting things away at work that I do once a day or week.			
I have a regular routine for putting things away at home that I do once a day or week.			
I file or delete my computer files when I am done with them.			
I have a regular routine for deleting files I don't need any more once a day or week.			
I don't buy or add items to my workspace or home unless I can give other things away.			

Continues…

Statement	Always	Sometimes	Rarely/Never
I value being organized because it makes me feel more productive.			
I value decluttering and minimizing unnecessary items in my workspace.			
I misplace items.			
I miss appointments because I forget them.			
I feel overwhelmed by the amount of clutter in my workspace.			
Subtotal per column	_____ x5	_____ x3	_____ x 1

Tally Your Score: Always = 5 points; Sometimes = 3 points; Rarely/Never = 1 point

Total Score: _____

46 to 60 points: You have effective organization skills. Continue practice time management and organization principles to maintain your ability.

30 to 45 points: You have some organization and decluttering skills, but there's room for improvement. Focus on the areas in which you can improve.

Below 29 points: Your life will feel less chaotic and more productive if you can begin practicing the following habits. Strive to address weaknesses in your skills by completing all of the activities.

This questionnaire was adapted from the article "How Good Is Your Time Management" by the Mind Tools Content Team. **https://SSPharm .ParadigmEducation.com/HowGood**

Getting Rid of Clutter

Studies show that having too much stuff, or clutter, can hamper your productivity and quality of life. **Clutter** consists of items that do not have an immediate use that gets in the way. It may be related to something you planned to do but never got around to, something someone gave you that you didn't want, or something you once used but no longer do. Clutter can also come from things that were once used, but not disposed of properly after you were done.

Now is the time to sort through and get rid of your clutter. Pick up each item, and ask yourself the following questions:

- Do I use it often? How often?
- Do I need or love it?
- Does it give me delight or make me laugh when I look at it or pick it up?

If you don't need or use it often and you don't love it, then it should be given away or discarded. Its usefulness to you is far less than the space it takes up. It gets in the way of your efficiency, productivity, and peace of mind.

If it is valuable in terms of sentiment or money, consider selling it. Or put the item in a pile to give away to friends or family or a donation center, so perhaps someone else can use it or find joy in it. Sentimental items are sometimes the hardest to part with, even if they serve no function. One tactic is to take a photo of the item for remembrance, which makes it easier to donate or give away. If it is useless, recycle the item or throw it away. If it is broken or unusable, put it into the trash. Once you have decluttered your space, don't bring anything into your organized area unless it will be used or loved. Consider practicing a one in, one out rule, and only purchase new items if they will replace something else. Do periodic checks to get rid of any clutter that made its way into your space.

> "If you don't need or use it often and you don't love it, then it should be given away or discarded."

Finding a Space for Everything

Once you have sorted your clutter, it is time to organize the essentials that are left. First, you will need to find homes for those items. Consider each space, starting with your workspace, and organize your computer in a similar way. Train yourself to always put each item back in the same place when you are done with it. This prevents a last-minute scramble to find things.

Determine the Purpose of the Space If you know the function of each part of your space, you can have a better idea of what belongs there. Keep only the things for that function or functions. Everything else should go.

Consider What Items Are Needed or Used Most Often Put these things in a tidy, organized way closest at hand. This can be accomplished by using a desk or drawer organizer, filing shelves, or whatever system works best for you.

Consider Less Often Accessed Items Put items that are important, but used less often, in a space not directly at hand but perhaps on a bookshelf nearby or in storage, depending upon the amount of use. If it is not used often, get it out of your immediate work area.

Organize Your Computer Files Keep documents used most often in easily accessed and organized files. The filing system should be understandable to others. Put any files that are not current into a well organized and easily found history file.

 Safety Alert

There is usually a "fast mover" shelf located near workstations in a pharmacy that holds the most commonly filled medications to increase efficiency. These need to be well organized, alphabetical by brand name or drug type so that the right drug is easy to locate without accidentally picking up a look-alike.

1.6 Module Summary

Developing the time-management skills used to meet deadlines and be productive takes practice. With continual effort, you'll find that creating well-organized to-do lists and planning your daily, weekly, and monthly activities becomes automatic. Stay focused and enjoy the feelings of relief and satisfaction as you check the tasks off your daily and weekly to-do lists. They will serve as your road maps to success.

You'll find that you build a sense of confidence as you make your appointments and meet deadlines. You will feel less stressed as you sit in an organized workspace and see yourself coming closer to achieving your short-term and long-term goals.

 The online course includes additional review and assessment resources.

Critical Thinking & Problem Solving

LEARNING OBJECTIVES

1 Understand critical thinking and its role in problem solving. (Section 2.1)

2 Identify the traits of a critical thinker. (Sections 2.1, 2.2)

3 Identify the behaviors of a critical thinker. (Sections 2.1, 2.2)

4 Learn the steps of effective problem solving. (Section 2.2)

5 Apply critical thinking and problem solving to workplace problems. (Section 2.2)

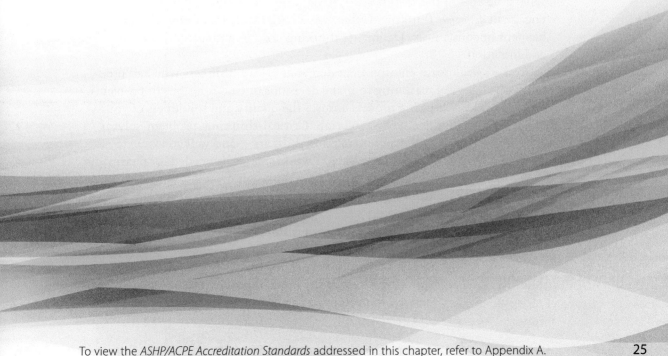

To view the *ASHP/ACPE Accreditation Standards* addressed in this chapter, refer to Appendix A.

The process of effective problem solving and critical thinking has many moving parts and can seem overwhelming. You must first stop and consider the question you are being asked. As you consider the problem, you engage in intentional and purposeful thought. Then, you apply the steps of effective problem solving to arrive at the answer. This process can be difficult when you are first learning it, like learning to drive a car. There are many steps to be aware of to operate an automobile and get from point A to point B. The process of driving, after a bit of practice, happens by reflex. With enough practice, the processes of critical thinking and problem solving will also become a reflex.

2.1 Critical Thinking

Critical thinking is the process of actively applying, analyzing, and evaluating information to form a well-reasoned judgment. Critical thinking evaluates all sides of an issue, action, or problem. Critical thinkers don't just accept an answer to a question but rather are curious about other possible conclusions or arguments. Analyzing all possible answers to a question leads to a clearer understanding of a subject, process, or belief. You have likely encountered the term *critical thinking* in your experience as a student. Educators use this term to describe thinking, learning, and analysis that go beyond the rote memorization and recall of facts.

Critical thinking is a crucial skill to learn for professional success. You will need this analytical reasoning to process information, make decisions, and solve problems in the workplace. Critical thinking requires you to pause and engage in *deliberate* thinking. Often, we do not think about how we think—it happens unconsciously. Deliberate thinking is done with careful consideration and intention.

Today's healthcare environment demands critical thinkers who can use purposeful, logical reasoning to make decisions or find solutions to problems. Using a critical-thinking process ensures the quality and soundness of your decision or solution. Critical-thinking, problem-solving, and decision-making skills are—and will continue to be—among the top workforce skills needed for pharmacy technicians. For that reason, you must know what critical thinking is and why it's important to learn and practice. It can be very easy to fall into patterns while on the job and complete tasks as if on autopilot. While many processes in the pharmacy are designed for redundancy and patient safety, they cannot be relied on by themselves. Critical thinking is one of the most important factors and the final defense to protecting the health and safety of our patients.

> "Critical thinking is one of the most important factors and the final defense to protecting the health and safety of our patients."

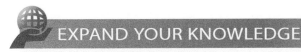

What are Employers Looking For?

A 2016 World Economic Forum report, *The Future of Jobs*, looks at the employment, skills, and workforce strategy for the future. The report asked chief human resources and strategy officers from leading global employers what the current shifts mean, specifically for employment, skills, and recruitment across industries and geographies. Complex problem solving, critical thinking, and judgment and decision-making are all on the top 10 list for workforce skills. To view the report, visit **https://SSPharm.ParadigmEducation.com/FutureJobs**.

This module will first identify the skills, traits, and processes of critical thinking, then apply the concepts to the process of problem solving. **Problem solving** is a systematic process for responding to a situation by crafting a solution. Problem solving is much more effective when critical thinking is used.

Understanding the Importance of Critical Thinking in Your Personal Life

Critical thinking is a crucial skill to learn for your personal life. You need analytical reasoning to process information, make decisions, and solve challenges that affect you and your family. Most of the thinking done daily is not deliberate and occurs automatically. For example, when you think about your daily routine, you might think of each of the steps that occur (making coffee, brushing your teeth, getting dressed, etc.), but you don't usually stop and carefully consider each step and why it is important. You simply think of what comes next and do that action. However, you might engage in critical thinking in other areas of your life, such as when you are weighing a large decision. For example, if you are considering moving to a new town, you'd carefully weigh your options, make lists of things that are important to you in a new city, research job openings in that area, and probably even ask yourself why you might want to move. When you apply critical thinking, you make better decisions that lead to better outcomes.

You have probably encountered critical thinking the most in your personal life as a student. Your instructors likely have given you assignments that go beyond simple recall and ask you to consider a scenario and how you would handle it. Critical thinking is a skill that increases academic success. If you can think critically about an essay question, for example, and form a well-reasoned response, you are more likely to get a high score. Good critical-thinking skills also illustrate to your instructors that you can apply what you have learned in class to the real world.

Understanding the Importance of Critical Thinking in the Workplace

The pharmacy setting is constantly evolving. It also has a high degree of variability. While the processes and general activities may remain the same, the challenges that arise within them are varied and require different approaches and solutions. There are many problems that occur with insurance plans, prescription clarifications, and customer interactions. This is where critical-thinking techniques are invaluable. Critical thinking is important to employers, the practice of pharmacy, and your career path.

Understand the Value to Employers Technicians who can think critically are better at adapting to different situations. These situations can include patient and physician interactions, workflow, and coworker relations. A pharmacy technician who applies critical thinking in the workplace is highly valued and considered much harder to replace than one who does not.

For example, when a technician can identify that a sign needs to be placed on the doors of the pharmacy announcing holiday operating times to prevent confusion, and the technician prints the sign before the pharmacist thinks of it, it is of immense value to an employer. Technicians who can think critically help keep the pharmacy running smoothly. When there is a line at the pharmacy counter of customers who have refill requests, some of which have issues with the third-party provider, you have to juggle processing the prescriptions and making phone calls to the insurance companies. When those third-party issues are complicated, you'll need to assess the various ways to handle them, all while communicating the issues to the patient and the pharmacist and handling your other assigned duties. Critical thinkers bring creative solutions to the workplace and think quickly on their feet, which are both skills that pharmacy employers value.

Understand the Value to Pharmacy Practice The ability to analyze processes and think about how they fit together in today's pharmacy allows for innovation and improvement. Critical thinkers can suggest new ways of doing things in the field, identify potential pitfalls in execution of initiatives, and help improve patient care. The field of pharmacy practice is constantly changing. New laws are enacted, new brand name drugs come to the market, generics become available for popular drugs, and technology evolves.

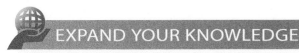

A Key Priority for Employers

A 2013 report of the Association of American Colleges and Universities, titled *It Takes More Than a Major: Employer Priorities for College Learning and Student Success*, summarized the findings of a national survey of business and nonprofit leaders.

The key findings of the report include the following:

- Nearly all employers surveyed (93%) say that "...a demonstrated capacity to think critically, communicate clearly, and solve complex problems is more important than [a candidate's] undergraduate major."
- Even more (95%) say they prioritize hiring college graduates with skills that will help

them contribute to innovation in the workplace.
- About 95% of those surveyed also say it is important that those they hire demonstrate ethical judgment and integrity; intercultural skills; and the capacity for continued new learning.
- More than 75% of those surveyed say they want more emphasis on five key areas, including critical thinking, complex problem solving, written communication, oral communication, and applied knowledge in real-world settings.

The report can be viewed at **https://SSPharm .ParadigmEducation.com/EmployerPriorities**.

Pharmacy technicians should always be ready to learn new skills, and they should be able to think critically about those skills.

Critical thinkers may ask why certain changes will improve the field. Considering why something is done the way that it is helps everyone to get on board with changes and may also point out areas that would benefit from a different approach. Critical thinkers assess new technology and not only adapt to using it but also think of other areas in which the technology could be applied or even improved. Successful pharmacy technicians can use critical-thinking skills to prioritize problems and make key decisions that improve patient care and even save lives.

Understand the Value to Your Career Path Many specialized roles that exist for technicians require critical-thinking skills to be successful. These roles involve higher authority, more complex activities, and increased compensation. Automation implementation specialists, technicians performing medication therapy management, and supervisors all regularly encounter challenges that use critical thinking to solve them effectively. In choosing where to apply your skills to further your career, critical thinking can be the factor between working in a setting that you can grow in and succeed or one that is stifling and not a proper fit. Critical thinking can be used to assess the culture and values of an employer to determine how well they align with your own personal values and work ethic.

Today's healthcare environment demands critical thinkers who can use purposeful, logical reasoning to make decisions or find solutions to problems. Using a critical-thinking process ensures the quality and soundness of your decision or solution. Almost all the interactions and tasks that can be done by a technician employ critical-thinking and problem-solving skills. For that reason, you need to know how to engage in the process of critical thinking. There are many traits and behaviors common to critical thinkers. Even if you do not currently possess these traits or behaviors, you can cultivate them to grow into a critical thinker.

Defining the Traits of an Effective Critical Thinker

Many studies and articles have shown which traits are necessary to develop to be an effective critical thinker. These include being a truth seeker, open minded, focused, curious, and many others. These traits can be improved to increase your critical-thinking abilities. The seven qualities listed below are hallmarks of effective critical thinkers.

Seek the Truth A technician who constantly verifies the information available based on facts, evidence, and reason is a seeker of truth. Statements are not taken at face value but supported with evidence-based research. Completing continuing education courses and reading pharmacy technology journals are behaviors that should be developed.

Have an Open Mind There are always two, if not more, viewpoints and sides to every story or situation. Elements such as prejudices, biases, and stereotypes can factor into these different perspectives, both in good and bad ways. A critical thinker considers all these elements and is willing to reconsider viewpoints as necessary.

Exhibit Analytical Reasoning When analyzing a problem or situation, a critical thinker tries to anticipate as many outcomes as possible, as well as arguments both for and against action on the situation or problem. This analysis prioritizes the problem and allows for it to be approached in the best manner.

Remain Organized and Focused To analyze effectively and ensure that all aspects of a situation or problem have been explored, being organized and having focus is required. Focus enables a critical thinker to concentrate on a subject through to its completion, while avoiding distractions and being organized allows for this focus to be applied to the necessary areas of a problem.

Practice Tip

In the community setting, it can be easy to assume things about patients who come into the pharmacy. You should not automatically think that someone is a narcotic drug seeker based on a first impression. Conversely, you cannot assume that patients are reputable just because they are clean-cut and polite.

Organize and Focus like a General

President Dwight D. Eisenhower created a method to stay focused and organize tasks that allowed him to complete numerous projects in a very efficient manner. Known as the "Eisenhower Matrix," it is a system to determine which action items need to be done first, scheduled for later, delegated to another person, or dropped completely. The matrix groups items by how important they are coupled with how quickly they need to be accomplished.

It can be very easy to lose focus and become disorganized, especially with projects that are long in duration or have many elements involved. Using this system can help maintain focus, and it uses many principles of critical thinking. More information can be found here: https://SSPharm.ParadigmEducation.com/EisenhowerMatrix.

Possess Self-Confidence Having self-confidence is what enables a critical thinker to trust in the analysis and course of action. Another aspect that involves self-confidence is the ability to admit when you are wrong or have made a mistake. Accountability can be considered a mark of self-confidence.

Display Curiosity A critical thinker constantly questions the way things operate in the workplace. Why does a process work or not work? Is there a better way to complete a task or innovate a process? If something is working very well, how can it be applied to other areas? Critical thinkers are willing to put forth the effort to implement changes where necessary or reinforce things that are beneficial.

Demonstrate Maturity Wisdom comes from both maturity and experience and is another trait of a critical thinker. The ability to think critically under pressure can be challenging, but maturity calms the emotions that impair the ability to find a solution to a problem. This experience does not have to come from the specific industry but from life in general.

 Think It Through: Are You a Critical Thinker?

Consider the traits of an effective thinker. Which traits do you currently possess? Which will take some effort on your part to cultivate?

Defining the Behaviors of an Effective Critical Thinker

Development of the traits for critical thinking is the first step in becoming an effective critical thinker. The next is to focus on the behaviors that promote critical thinking. These behaviors include recognizing problems, communicating and collaborating, analyzing, asking the right questions, and many others. By being aware and focusing on the actions and thought processes listed below, critical thinking becomes a more routine action in your interactions both personally and professionally.

Recognize Problems to Solve or Decisions to Be Made Sometimes employees do not even recognize there is a problem, either with themselves or with the process they are performing. This lack of awareness does not exist with critical thinkers, as they are constantly analyzing their work and environment to assess effectiveness.

Communicate and Collaborate Effectively Thinking about a problem or process is the first step; articulating it and collaborating is the second. Being able to clearly express what your critical thinking has uncovered and working together with your coworkers and supervisors is essential to being able to address the situation.

Analyze the Relevance and Validity of Information When discovering information on a subject or situation, there may be a large amount to sift through. A critical thinker knows how to determine the relevance and authenticity of the various data points. This allows them to use the pertinent information to reach a decision or solve the problem.

Ask Vital Questions The curiosity trait discussed previously leads to questioning. Asking the *right* questions is a behavior of a person who thinks critically. Effective questioning not only identifies problems and solutions, it can also determine if a question needs to be asked in the first place. The questions that a reporter or author asks when writing a story, are the foundation to build their stories. They are commonly known as the "five Ws and H"—who, what, where, when, why, and how. Table 2.1 illustrates some examples of how the five Ws and H can be applied. These are general statements but are adaptable to patient interactions, analysis of a process in an institutional setting, coworker dynamics, etc.

Regulate Emotions It can be easy to let emotions have control over actions, especially in high-stress situations or interactions. Reacting to the emotions of others, while natural, is not the strategy of a critical thinker and problem solver. Regulating emotions by being proactive and analytical is a behavior that critical thinkers exhibit.

Table 2.1 The Five Ws and H	
Who	…will benefit/not benefit from this decision?
	…might need to be informed or consulted regarding the problem or decision?
	…can you ask for help, if necessary?
What	…is the purpose of addressing this problem?
	…are the pros and cons of the potential solution or decision?
	…is another perspective considered when addressing the problem?
	…is another approach to the problem?
	…is the best/worst outcome of the decision or action?
	…are the challenges to solving this?
	…are situations you can use for comparison?
Where	…can you gather more information?
	…is the area that needs most improvement?
When	…is the best time to implement the solution or decision?
	…should you ask for assistance solving this problem?
Why	…is this problem or decision requiring action?
	…should others be informed about this problem?
	…has this problem not been addressed prior?
	…is this solution or action necessary?
How	…does this problem or decision affect operations?
	…does this affect you or others in the pharmacy?
	…can you solve this problem?

Connect Pieces of Information to Find a Combined Meaning Finding and understanding various pieces of information that surround a subject is not enough for critical thinking to apply. These pieces of information must be compared to each other to identify cause-and-effect relationships and the bigger picture in general.

Consider a Solution, Decision, or Conclusion Once a decision is reached based on careful analysis, connections, etc., thought must also be dedicated to that decision or solution. Weighing the pros and cons or outcomes of a potential decision is an important part of critical thinking. Many times, people make a decision without considering the consequences, and the solution does not work out as well as it could have.

Self-Reflection:
How Would You Gauge Your Critical-Thinking Skills?

Read each statement. If you feel confident that you can say "yes" to that statement, place a check mark in the first column. Respond to statements as honestly as possible.

✔	Statement
	I make a logical plan of action.
	I discern a fact from an opinion.
	I examine a problem from different perspectives.
	I recognize bias, stereotyping, and prejudice in information I read.
	I evaluate the merits of an argument or line of reasoning.
	I control my emotions when making an argument or a decision.
	I concede to others when I am wrong.
	I identify inconsistencies or errors in reasoning.
	I approach problems or decisions in a systemic, organized manner.
	I identify resources to help me solve a problem or make a decision.
	I collaborate with others to find a solution or make a decision.
	I ask questions to gain insight into the thinking of others.
	I remain motivated when trying to solve a problem or make a decision.

Tally Your Score: One check mark = 1 point

Total Score: _____

10 to 13 points: This score indicates you have excellent critical-thinking skills.

6 to 9 points: This score indicates that you sometimes exhibit the behavior of a critical thinker but could improve in this area.

Below 6 points: This score indicates that you do not behave like a critical thinker and need to develop your skills.

2.2 Problem Solving

While critical thinking tends to focus on long-term planning, problems, and scenarios, the behaviors and traits used are also the tools employed to solve shorter-term individual problems, which are an everyday occurrence for pharmacy technicians. As stated earlier, problem solving is the systematic process for responding to a situation by crafting a solution. There are different systems that can be used to solve problems effectively, but most employ similar strategies. By learning a system and using it consistently, a solution can be found for most problems encountered with a minimum amount of difficulty.

Learning more about a problem is the primary way in which to solve it. The steps that are taken include identification, understanding, application, and analysis. These steps are modeled after those in Bloom's Taxonomy. **Bloom's Taxonomy** is a set of principles and hierarchies that classify the process of learning, which you may have encountered in your pharmacy technician education. The levels in Bloom's Taxonomy are Remember, Understand, Apply, Analyze, Evaluate, and Create. Figure 2.1 illustrates the levels in Bloom's Taxonomy.

Figure 2.1 Bloom's Taxonomy

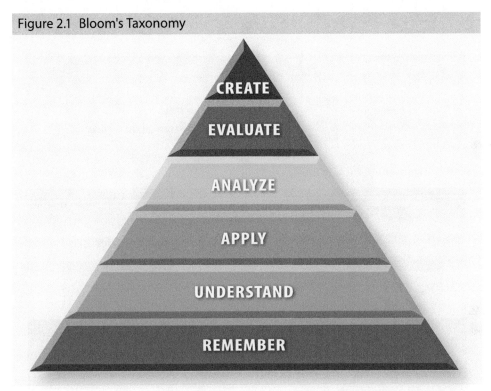

The steps listed below can be used to solve problems both short and long term by using critical thinking behaviors and traits:

- identify a decision that needs to be made, an issue that needs to be addressed, a problem that needs to be solved, or a course of action that needs to be taken
- seek information to clarify and better understand the decision, issue, problem, or course of action
- formulate a potential decision, solution, conclusion, or course of action
- consider the pros and cons of the decision, solution, conclusion, or course of action
- arrive at the best decision, solution, conclusion, or course of action

The steps involved in problem solving use the behaviors and traits belonging to effective critical thinkers, as shown in Figure 2.2.

Figure 2.2 Effective Critical Thinkers

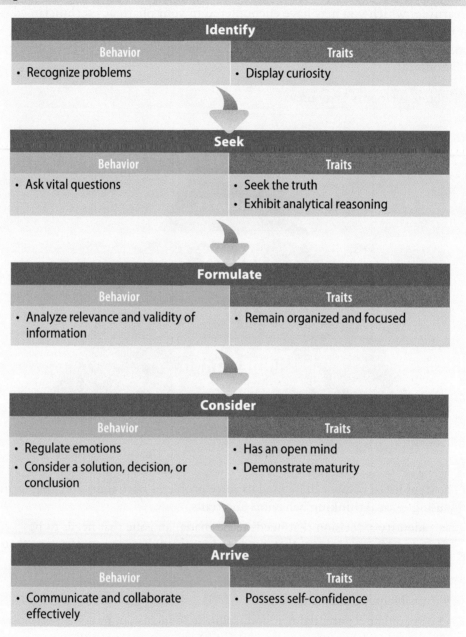

Identify	
Behavior	**Traits**
• Recognize problems	• Display curiosity

Seek	
Behavior	**Traits**
• Ask vital questions	• Seek the truth
	• Exhibit analytical reasoning

Formulate	
Behavior	**Traits**
• Analyze relevance and validity of information	• Remain organized and focused

Consider	
Behavior	**Traits**
• Regulate emotions	• Has an open mind
• Consider a solution, decision, or conclusion	• Demonstrate maturity

Arrive	
Behavior	**Traits**
• Communicate and collaborate effectively	• Possess self-confidence

As we go more in-depth into the problem-solving steps, we will examine a scenario from the field as a reference and apply the steps to solve the problem.

The scenario: Several instances of suspected anthrax exposures due to bioterrorism have led some nurses to stockpile Levaquin by using diversion. You are the automation technician in charge of Pyxis operations. How would you proceed?

Identifying the Problem

Identification of a problem involves several steps. Not following steps can lead to impulsive reactions or acting under less-than–optimal conditions. A complaint from a doctor about a pharmacy policy should not lead to an immediate changing of the policy, which can affect multiple departments. While speed may be of the essence, it should not supersede analysis of the issue. These steps can be followed rapidly, but all of them should be followed to come to an accurate understanding of the problem. Articulating or defining the issue, deciding why it is important to address, and making observations of the situation lead to proper identification of a problem.

Define the Problem What is the problem you want to solve? How can you use your knowledge/experience to address this problem? At this point, you must not define the problem in terms of the solution—just define the problem itself.

In the example scenario, the problem to be solved is nurses diverting Levaquin within the hospital. This is occurring after a rash of anthrax-laced letters was discovered being sent throughout the country. As the automation technician, you have the knowledge of how Levaquin is dispensed on the nursing floors and the access to fix the problem.

Recognize the Motivation for Solving the Problem If there is a legitimate need to solve the problem, then the effort put forth to do so is worth it. Part of identification is to determine if the problem is in fact serious enough to merit further actions. Sometimes you may find that solving a problem is not worth the hassle.

In the case of the diversion, there is a need. Levaquin is an expensive medication, and the effort to keep it in stock for patients who need it, not to mention the extra phone calls that must be made when it is out of stock, justifies solving the problem. There are also ethical issues involved in drug diversion, further warranting that the problem be solved.

Make Observations Observing ties back to the process of questioning. You must step back and make careful observations and ask key questions. Who is

Practice Tip

If you are trying to find motivation to solve a problem in your pharmacy, one question to ask includes, "Will this benefit myself, the department, or the company?" If the answer is yes to any of these, then you have found the motivation.

involved in the problem? How often does the problem occur? When did the problem start? Where does it occur?

> In the example scenario, the Pharmacy and the Nursing Departments are involved with the problem. The problem is encountered during every fill of the Pyxis machines, and it started once media attention focused on the threat of anthrax poisoning and the public became aware of the potential risk. Review of reports from the Pyxis reveal that the diversion is most likely occurring in three of the eight nursing units in the facility.

Seeking to Understand the Problem

Understanding the problem in its entirety can happen in conjunction with identification. The steps involved in understanding will lead to the next steps of the problem-solving process. It will also help in articulating the problem to coworkers and supervisors. Many problems encountered are not solved in a vacuum, and enlisting the aid of others is necessary. The more you understand the problem, the better you can express its significance to others. Full understanding comes from being able to state a problem's scope and root cause. Identifying how others view the problem and gathering as much available information about the problem leads to complete understanding.

Identify Its Scope and Significance Once you know the nature of a problem, you can assess its significance. This is also known as *triaging*. How large is the problem? How significant is it? Should addressing this problem be a priority?

> The diversion scenario is very significant, and while perhaps not institutionwide, it affects a significant portion of the institution and several departments.

Determine Its Root Cause The root of a problem is not always immediately clear and may be interpreted differently by people with different perspectives on the situation. Determining why it is a problem is part of determining its root cause and ultimately its solution.

> The root cause of the example scenario is fear of anthrax poisoning. It is a problem due to the high cost of the missing medication, but more importantly, its diversion is potentially affecting care to patients who already have an infection and have been prescribed the medication.

Recognize Others' Perspectives To enlist the aid of others, as mentioned above, it is important to assess the perspectives of all parties involved. How do they feel about this problem? What experiences have they had with this problem? How did they try to solve this problem, if at all?

In the example scenario, one must consider the perspectives of other technicians and pharmacy staff. The buyer is upset at having to order extra Levaquin, as it puts the department over its budget. The central technician is annoyed at having to field extra calls about missing doses of the medication. Nursing administration does not consider it as great a problem and is worried about other areas of care. The nursing units in question do not want to admit that some of their staff may be stealing medication.

Gather Information The more information you have about the situation, or those like it, the better you can solve or address it. "Don't reinvent the wheel" is a saying that exists for a very good reason. If there is a protocol or solution that someone else has applied to the problem, perhaps in another setting or a different but similar scenario, that can be used for the existing problem. Conferring with experienced individuals and conducting independent research and fact finding are methods to gather information.

In the example, pulling reports on inventory discrepancies, researching control mechanisms for diversion, and talking with pharmacy leadership are all methods of gathering information.

Formulating and Applying Your Gathered Information to the Problem

By synthesizing the information gathered and using it for further analysis, options for resolution start to become available. This synthesis occurs by organizing the data found and making sure that it is reliable and valid. Having organized data will also allow you to begin to see patterns in the information. Identifying patterns can help you develop a solution.

Organize the Information Organizing will not only allow you to process all the data obtained but also enable you to present a coherent picture of the problem to those who need to be made aware of it. Coworkers and supervisors appreciate an organized, concise appraisal of a situation.

With the example scenario, you must organize the reports of access to the medication and cost in excess ordering and gather data regarding similar diversion scenarios. Organizing this information can also help identify if there is any information missing that needs to be obtained before moving forward.

Determine Reliability and Validity of the Information When researching a problem, some of the data may not be reliable and must be discarded. If the source is not reliable, the data is not valid.

Fortunately, reporting systems in automation are very accurate and reliable, if employees are using them properly. In this case, it would be prudent to check to see if there were any incidences of human error, such as improper filling of the Pyxis machine.

Observe Patterns in the Information When information is gathered and organized efficiently, it is much easier to analyze it for patterns or trends. Disorganized data can be taken out of context and can be essentially worthless.

For the Levaquin scenario, the reports generated are very effective at showing patterns in the use and access to the medication. Specific units and nurses can be looked at to determine if there are patterns or correlations between missing stock and their access to the medication.

Considering and Analyzing Potential Solutions

By understanding the nature of a problem, the data involved, and the patterns inherent in them, possible solutions can be crafted and examined for viability. Ways to examine solutions include brainstorming different paths that can be taken and then weighing the pros and cons for each option.

In the Levaquin scenario, since the data points to specific units and nurses for access, the potential solutions can be to restrict access for those particular nurses, those units, or the entire institution.

Brainstorm Solutions In a field such as pharmacy, there is typically more than one method or solution to a given problem. Brainstorming different ways to solve a problem ensures that there are a variety of solutions to choose from. The first idea is not always the best one. However, if it is the best idea, that is verified by exploring all possible alternatives.

While restriction of access is the first option that came to mind, it may not be the only one available. Since the diversion is a result of fear of anthrax, education is a potential remedy. Perhaps a training session with the specific departments on the nature of anthrax poisonings and bioterrorism statistics can help alleviate the fear. Another question that needs to be answered is, if access restriction is chosen, what is the best way to restrict access? Should the drug be hand delivered from the pharmacy? Should the drug be classified as a controlled substance and loaded into the Pyxis machine with the same control mechanisms as a CII medication?

Assess the Strengths and Weaknesses of Each Solution Potential solutions to problems have consequences when implemented and must be considered carefully when choosing a course of action. A pros and cons list is very useful in assessing available options.

In the institutional scenario, the pro of controlling access to Levaquin is that it will be much more difficult to divert, as there is a count taken every time it is accessed. Restriction would prevent excess ordering and allow the pharmacy to stay under budget with the weekly and monthly drug orders. The cons are that it would take longer for nurses to get this medication for dispensing and for the technician to load it into the Pyxis machine. This delay has the potential to increase frustrations in both departments.

Arriving at an Action Plan

Once a solution is decided upon, it must be examined in further detail before being put into use. The more comprehensive the examination, the more likely the solution will be effective.

Creating an action plan is the final step to engage in solving a problem. It is an organized checklist of steps that are accomplished to complete the solution. Depending on the scope of the solution, this could be quite detailed or as small as a bulleted list of items. It is very useful for summarizing the solution and ensuring that all parties involved understand what is being done about the problem.

An action plan for the example scenario would be to have timelines for training and implementation of the new process, checklists of key personnel and departments involved and their roles, and a plan for follow-up and review of the process. An example of the action plan for the Levaquin scenario is illustrated in Figure 2.3

Figure 2.3 Sample Action Plan

Task	Timeline	Key Personnel	Follow-Up
Add restrictions to Pyxis machine	Immediately	Pyxis Technician, Pharmacy Department	Pharmacy Department to test restrictions
Train Pharmacy Department on new Pyxis procedures	Within one week	Pharmacy Department	Pharmacy Department to train all technicians
Train Nursing Department on new Pyxis procedures	Within two weeks	Pharmacy Department, Nursing Department	Pharmacy Department to train the Nursing Department. Nursing Department will follow up with superiors to ensure all have gone through the training
All hospital staff training on anthrax and bioterrorism	Within one month	All hospital staff	All staff will receive certification of training

Identify Barriers to Implementing the Solution By determining potential barriers to using a solution, they can be avoided entirely. Identifying barriers will also help you figure out the best way to implement a solution. Things that should be addressed include time constraints, budget, resources, and training.

For the anthrax situation, lack of understanding for the new process and nursing compliance are barriers. A training plan with the nursing and pharmacy departments should be developed that explains the situation, the need for control, and the process being implemented.

Monitor the Progress of the Action Plan It is true that no plan survives first contact with the enemy. Whether in sports, war, or work, variables are always in play, and even the most well-laid plans need adjustment and modification. Follow–up is key to ensuring a solution works. Is the action plan on track? Are changes needed in the plan? Is the solution successful?

For the Levaquin protocol, follow-up reviews were set for 30, 60, and 90 days after implementation. Inventory numbers would be checked to determine effectiveness, and staff would be surveyed to assess mood and compliance with the process, as well as address any questions or concerns.

> ### Think It Through: Additional Problem Solving Activities
> Review the sample critical-thinking scenarios in the online courseware that require the problem-solving skills discussed in this module. What would be the potential workflow for the situation, and how would you apply problem-solving skills you have learned?

2.3 Module Summary

Critical thinking is a valuable skill that can be used both personally and in the pharmacy setting. By exhibiting the right traits and practicing certain behaviors, you will improve your ability to think critically. Problem solving is a skill that uses critical thinking to systematically come up with a solution to a situation. There will be many chances to engage critical-thinking skills in your career as a pharmacy technician. Critical thinking and problem solving go hand in hand. These abilities, when properly honed, will make you a valuable employee to any pharmacy.

 The online course includes additional review and assessment resources.

Professional Appearance

LEARNING OBJECTIVES

1 Explain the importance of first impressions. (Section 3.1)

2 Identify the meaning and importance of a professional image in the pharmacy. (Section 3.1)

3 Identify the professional appearance expectations for pharmacy technicians. (Section 3.2)

4 Identify examples of the impact of appearance on your career as a pharmacy technician. (Section 3.2)

5 Identify your hygiene needs and standards. (Section 3.2)

6 Dress appropriately for different pharmacy settings. (Section 3.2)

7 Demonstrate professional eye contact and facial expression. (Section 3.3)

8 Recognize proper posture and its importance for professional appearance. (Section 3.3)

To view the *ASHP/ACPE Accreditation Standards* addressed in this chapter, refer to Appendix A.

A wareness of your everyday appearance and hygiene is necessary for career success. These are the first qualities that your future employers will likely observe about you in your interview for employment or while on externship. Employees are expected to represent not only themselves but also their employers and their professions. This expectation is true for most jobs. Dressing and presenting yourself in a manner that aligns with employer standards will help to ensure that your knowledge and skills are the qualities that others remember.

Understanding how to dress and groom appropriately for a position is a necessary skill for anyone looking for work or hoping to advance in a career. This module describes the purpose of cultivating a professional image and identifies how you can improve your professional appearance before you enter the workforce, including how well you dress and groom, how you carry yourself, and what impression your appearance creates.

3.1 Professional Image

Work Wise

Personal and professional images may not always align. Be prepared to adjust your personal style for interview and employment situations.

The way you look and carry yourself helps to create your professional image. For our purposes, **image** describes the way that you present yourself to others by your choice in clothing, behavior, communication style, body language, and hygiene. A **professional image** describes the way you present yourself while at work, while representing your employer, or while seeking employment. A professional image considers the expectations of the industry and the employer as well as the relationships and interactions you may have with customers, patients, colleagues, and supervisors.

These relationships and expectations should be considered when you cultivate your image. The image you create will produce an instant first impression—that is, its visual impact—on others and will either be a benefit or a hinderance to your success. Other elements of professional image (e.g., behavior, interpersonal interactions, and courtesies) are discussed in Module 4.

Creating a Professional Image in the Workplace

As you create your professional image, keep a few things in mind: The choices you make related to your image will affect several areas in your daily interactions and future success. The image you create can influence your own self-perception and can also affect how others view you and your abilities. For this reason, your self-perception, the way others perceive you, and the resulting impression can affect many levels in your career.

To gauge your own self-perception, take the following self-reflection and consider which areas could be improved or reinforced.

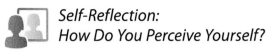

Self-Reflection:
How Do You Perceive Yourself?

For each statement, answer "always," "sometimes," or "rarely." Respond to statements as honestly as possible.

When considering my own personal traits, I...	Always	Sometimes	Rarely
feel confident.			
am comfortable in my own skin.			
take pride in my appearance.			
believe I have strengths.			
understand my weaknesses.			
do not compare myself to others.			
reflect on experiences and their effects in my life.			
reflect on choices I have made and their effects in my life.			
Subtotal per column	_____ x5	_____ x3	_____ x1

Tally Your Score: Always = 5 points; Sometimes = 3 points; Rarely = 1 point

Total Score: _____

31 to 40 points: You have a strong self-perception.

26 to 30 points: Your self-perception is satisfactory but could be improved.

16 to 25 points: Your self-perception has areas that can be worked on for improvement.

Below 16 points: Your self-perception is more negative than positive and could be improved. Consider what you might do to improve these areas.

Creating a Positive First Impression

If you search for "professional image" or "career advancement," you'll find a number of articles and career advisers offering advice on how to create a positive first impression. Scientific studies continue to find that first impressions happen within seven seconds or less, which is especially important when you interview for a new job or meet new colleagues.

In the pharmacy profession, technicians are the initial point of contact in any setting. In the hospital and community pharmacy setting, you are the first and often last person patients or nurses see when they are filling prescriptions. Almost all telephone interactions are first initiated or received by a technician. The professional image you project will set the tone for all future interactions with a given provider or patient.

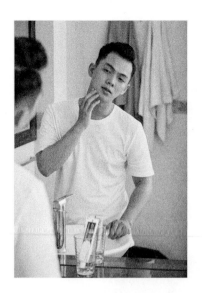

Your physical appearance is the first thing that people observe when they meet you. They will notice how you are dressed and groomed, as well as your facial expressions, gestures, and posture. These nonverbal cues make an impression on whomever you encounter. They can convey confidence, professionalism, and competence—or if not managed appropriately, the exact opposite.

As a pharmacy technician, the messages you convey to customers in your body posture, facial expressions, and demeanor reflect both you and your employer. Understanding your employer's goals and the expectations of your profession will help you create the type of image you need to present to succeed in the pharmacy. Every message you display (whether verbal or nonverbal) can be observed by others and should be factored into your assessment of your own professional image.

3.2 Personal and Professional Appearance

Your **personal appearance** describes your choices in personal hygiene, grooming, clothing, and body adornment (e.g., jewelry, piercings, and tattoos) in your personal life. These choices will either help or hinder your professional image. They leave an impression on others, such as potential employers, coworkers, and customers; so respect the importance of these choices as you leave the training environment and move into the workforce.

It is important to be able to meet the expectations of the industry for grooming and appearance whenever necessary. Personal appearance choices that do not align are not prohibited outside of work, but you must be able to adopt a professional image while on duty. **Professional appearance** is the way you dress, groom, and carry yourself while at your place of employment, and includes not only wearing appropriate clothing, but practicing proper hygiene. Assessing your current personal and professional appearance will allow you to better identify how you can improve in these areas.

Think It Through: Assess Your Appearance

Think about your current clothing and grooming practices—specifically what you engaged in when you last left your house. If you had to introduce yourself to a prospective employer right now, how might the person describe your appearance? What impression might you make on a stranger? Would you have wanted to make any changes to your appearance before interacting with a prospective employer? If so, what would they be?

Adjusting Your Appearance from Student to Pharmacy Professional

Although your appearance and hygiene do not affect your ability to learn the course material itself, your transition from student to pharmacy professional will begin before you complete your program. Many schools and technician programs have dress codes and professionalism rubrics that can affect your grade. These efforts help to instill and encourage professional appearance behaviors before graduation and will help you transition into the workforce quickly.

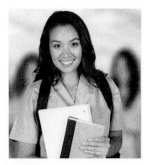

Pharmacy technician students may need to adjust their appearance to meet the requirements of local employers.

The ability to cultivate a professional appearance is essential to your success. The choices you make related to your appearance can mean the difference between obtaining and succeeding in a job, and not getting past the first interview.

An externship may be considered an extended working job interview. When you meet with your externship mentor and begin your rotation, you will be expected to dress the part of a full-time pharmacy technician. To begin to get an idea of what this entails, a simple Google image search of "pharmacy technicians" will return many examples of professional dress and appearance. To help gauge your self-awareness, refer to the Self-Reflection activity below.

Self-Reflection: How Do You Prepare for Your Day?

For each statement, answer "always," "sometimes," or "rarely." Respond to statements as honestly as possible.

When preparing for my day, I...	Always	Sometimes	Rarely
bathe or shower.			
use deodorant.			
avoid strong-smelling perfume or cologne.			
keep my hair clean and groomed.			
make sure my fingernails are clean and trimmed.			
brush my teeth.			
wear clothing that is conservative in style.			
wear clean clothing free of wrinkles.			
wear clothing that fits comfortably and appropriately.			
wear clothing that is free from tears, rips, and stains.			
choose clothing and jewelry that align with the pharmacy technician industry.			
Subtotal per column	_____ x5	_____ x3	_____ x1

Continues…

Tally Your Score: Always = 5 points; Sometimes = 3 points; Rarely = 1 point

Total Score:_____

45 to 55 points: There is little area for improvement in your professional appearance.

35 to 44 points: Your current level of professional appearance is satisfactory but could be improved.

25 to 34 points: Your professional appearance and grooming practices could be improved.

Below 25 points: Your professional appearance and grooming practices do not meet the standards of your industry, and you should work quickly and diligently to address your choices.

Think It Through: Self-Expression

It can be difficult for some people to balance the expectations of their employer with their own needs of self-expression and self-perception. Your overall appearance and attire can affect your mood, health, confidence, self-esteem, and productivity. Consider the last time you had to wear something that didn't align with your personal preferences. It's likely that you didn't feel comfortable and were perhaps distracted by your discomfort. Consider the challenges you might face as you build your professional image for your externship, job interviews, and future job.

Practice Tip

Scents from perfumes, body washes, and other products are unique because they can be equally acceptable and unacceptable to different people. In the workplace, it is best to assume that a fragrance-free environment is preferred.

Adopting Good Personal Hygiene

Although wardrobe choices are a key part of developing a professional appearance, professional clothing or accessories cannot make up for poor hygiene. An ill-fitting jacket or shirt could be overlooked, but an unpleasant smell (whether body odor or perfume) is more likely to not be ignored. Unpleasant smells could be related to hygiene choices (failing to bathe regularly or brushing your teeth after eating) or grooming choices (wearing strong perfumes or cologne). Maintaining good personal hygiene is an expectation you'll find across nearly every industry.

You've just self-reflected on your own personal hygiene and where you might improve. The next step will be to identify and maintain these hygiene practices and then recognize their impact in the pharmacy.

Maintain Hygiene Practices All pharmacies expect their employees to follow basic personal hygiene practices. There are even more stringent requirements for various medication preparations (such as hazardous or sterile preparations). Basic hygiene rules include the following:

- Shower or bathe daily.
- Brush your teeth daily.
- Use deodorant daily.
- Wash your hands thoroughly after every trip to the restroom.
- Keep your hair clean and styled neatly. In some pharmacy settings, fad hairstyles and unnatural hair colors may not be allowed, especially if you are expected to interact with the public.
- Keep your fingernails clean and trimmed.
- Trim and groom facial hair.
- Avoid using products that have a strong fragrance. Use perfume or cologne sparingly (if at all). Some companies are scent free and do not allow you to wear perfume or cologne in the workplace.
- Use mouthwash and/or breath mints after every cigarette (if you smoke).

 Work Wise

Cigarette smoke lingers on your clothing, and others may find this unprofessional. Take care to ensure that the clothes you wear to work are relatively odor free. Febreze or other fabric deodorizers can be especially useful.

WORKPLACE WISDOM

Fashion in the Pharmacy

As an instructor, I have encountered the occasional argument that certain clothing or hairstyles should be accepted in the workplace. Students have argued that dress codes are old-fashioned or too strict and fail to allow current trends or styles. My response is that the pharmacy likely considered a number of factors when establishing the dress code—including whether the customer demographic would be more at ease with employees in conservative dress. The pharmacy and its employees must be aware of standards and norms for its entire population to retain customers.

–Mark Brunton, MSHE, CPhT

Recognize the Impact of Hygiene in the Workplace Hygiene practices are important for any profession, but working in a pharmacy requires additional consideration in relation to hygiene. Behind the counter, you will be handling the medication that will be ingested by your patient. Much like food prep workers, we must have the same considerations for hygiene. You will also be one of the first people with whom the customer engages. The customer may have a weaker immune system, and maintaining cleanliness helps to prevent the spread of illness in both directions. Your proper hygiene and grooming choices will ensure that your colleagues and customers can interact with you without hindrance.

Work Environment All members of the pharmacy team need to be able to focus on their work and get along relatively well while doing so. Consider also that pharmacies can be in a small space, with employees working in very close proximity. Medication errors can occur from the smallest distractions. Body odor, heavy fragrances, or other poor hygiene choices can disrupt the processes involved in dispensing and can cause others to focus poorly on their tasks. These are avoidable distractions and must be considered daily.

Workplace Relationships As a pharmacy technician, you will interact with many people and develop relationships with pharmacists, other technicians, and customers. These interactions should be pleasant and you are expected to ensure that your hygiene does not negatively affect others. Customers picking up medications or consulting with a pharmacist may be ill (or caring for someone who is ill), and they depend on you and other health professionals to help prevent the spread of infection or not exacerbate their conditions.

Employment Jeopardy Employees who do not follow the company policies for hygiene are at risk for receiving the same disciplinary measures that are possible for other policy violations, such as tardiness and insubordination. These can include verbal and written warnings, probations, and suspensions, up to and including termination from the company.

Donning Professional Apparel

The first step in determining how to dress for work is finding out what the dress code is for your pharmacy. A **dress code** is a policy that describes the standard of acceptable attire and grooming in a specific workplace. This policy will usually be addressed during orientation after employment or before externship. The dress code typically addresses a range of appearance issues, such as required attire, uniforms, shoes, jewelry, makeup, body art, and—in some workplaces—hairstyles.

Pharmacists may create dress code policies to ensure a unified professional appearance and to protect the health and safety of employees and customers. For instance, there is no makeup allowed while compounding sterile preparations, as it can contaminate the product. Sometimes scrubs or business casual are acceptable attire. This promotes patient trust in the pharmacy as healthcare professionals who will handle their prescriptions safely. Scrubs are standard attire in hospital settings.

Know Your Facility's Dress Code Nearly every pharmacy has a dress code. It may be a uniform or uniform smock, scrubs, or business casual attire depending on the setting or employer. Invest in two or more uniforms or outfits to clean and rotate. Scrubs can be purchased both online and at local uniform stores.

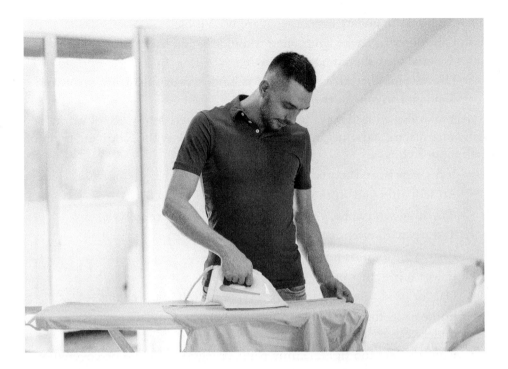

For pharmacies that allow business casual attire, it is always best to err on the side of caution (more formal vs. less). Regardless of the type of uniform, articles must always be clean and wrinkle free before use.

For business casual footwear, wear dress shoes or low heeled or flat shoes. Closed-toe shoes are mandatory for safety. In a hospital setting, sneakers are often allowed, provided they are kept clean and presentable. Note that, regardless of style, shoes should be comfortable to wear for long periods while standing, providing both cushion and support. Technicians rarely sit while working and may be off of their feet only during lunches and breaks.

When not assigned a specific uniform—or when interviewing for a position—it is best to wear clothing that meets the following standards:

- Button-down shirts (perhaps with a tie for men) or collared shirts (shirts should always be tucked in, unless it is a long top or sweater meant to cover pants or skirts)
- Dress pants or slacks that fit properly
- A belt that matches shoe color
- Socks that match pant or shoe color
- Closed-toe shoes that are comfortable for standing for long periods of time, with an appropriate heel height (under two inches) and in good condition

 Safety Alert

When working in a pharmacy, it is not uncommon for items to roll or fall off countertops. A common instinct is to "catch" them with your foot to slow their fall. This reaction is sometimes referred to as "pharmacist foot." Things like glass bottles, ampules, or needles could injure you if you don't wear closed-toed shoes.

- Appropriate undergarments that are not visible
- Clothing that covers your chest, shoulders, and back (cleavage or exposed back should not be shown)
- Dresses and skirts that are at least as long as your fingertips when your hands are at your sides

You may also wish to consider what not to wear to your place of work. Many pharmacies and other businesses would not allow the following types of clothing or styling:

- Jeans, capris, and shorts
- Athletic suits and workout gear
- Anything with holes, rips, or frays (even if they are in style)
- T-shirts with offensive language or images
- Pajama bottoms or tops
- Revealing clothes of any kind
- Hats or head coverings indoors, except for religious reasons
- Loose pants that need to be pulled up constantly or that expose underwear
- Pants that are too tight; skinny pants or leggings should be covered by a long top or sweater
- Flip-flops, open-toed sandals, and high heels

Although many pharmacies require employees to wear a specific uniform, you may find that some pharmacies allow more casual dress. Khakis, jeans, and even capris may be permitted. This trend is seen more in closed-door and mail-order settings. If this is the case, you can adjust your work wardrobe accordingly. However, it is best to overdress for your externship and for your first days of any job rather than to underdress; then you can adjust your wardrobe based on the employer's standards.

Work Wise

Dressing more formally can increase your sense of confidence and remind you of your professional status and competence.

WORKPLACE WISDOM

Perfecting Pharmacy Attire

When selecting your wardrobe to fit the dress code, choose fabrics that wear well. Cotton, while comfortable, fades and gets worn out quickly. Typically, a polyester, rayon, or polyester/cotton blend will last longer. These fabrics also are more wrinkle resistant and need less maintenance. Be sure to choose items that fit comfortably and are not too tight or too baggy.

Know Your Facility's Rules Regarding Body Adornment Pharmacies and hospital health systems and institutions have values, mission statements, and an overall impression they wish to convey to patients and the community in general. Body adornments, which can be considered stylish or trendy, may not align with these goals. Your pharmacy's dress code will dictate the rules of wearing and displaying body adornment, such as jewelry (including piercings) or tattoos. Different facilities may have different expectations related to body adornment, but note that in sterile compounding, jewelry is not permitted at all.

Work Wise

The sterile compounding environment is the strictest area with regard to body adornment.

Facial Piercings In most cases, avoid wearing excessive ear or facial piercings. Most policies will state that body and facial piercing of any kind should not be visible, and large-gauge earrings may require a flesh-colored plug while on duty.

Jewelry Avoid flashy, large jewelry and a large amount of them. One or two pieces is enough. A ring and a necklace or a watch and a ring are examples of moderate items for accessorizing.

Visible Tattoos Visible tattoos may or may not be allowed in your facility. If they are not, invest in makeup or clothing that will conceal or cover your tattoos.

Know Your Facility's Rules Regarding Grooming Grooming standards for the pharmacy setting are designed to maintain the necessary degree of cleanliness for healthcare environments, whether it be in a clean room or at a prescription drop-off window. They are meant to convey a neat, approachable, and trust-inspiring image for patients. These standards can apply to hair, makeup, and fragrances.

Hair Color and Hair Accessories Any facial hair should be trimmed and well-groomed (including nose and ear hair). If working in a sterile environment, covers for facial hair, such as surgical masks, are necessary.

Natural hair colors are the safest choice when starting out in the pharmacy (unless the pharmacy has a policy that color does not matter if hair is properly groomed).

Makeup As mentioned previously, makeup is prohibited in a sterile compounding environment to prevent contamination of a sterile preparation. When not working in the sterile compounding environment, makeup may be worn. One might recommend that an intern or job applicant wear makeup that is natural in appearance, without excessive eye or lip color. This guideline may be adjusted as an employee begins to understand the grooming expectations of their particular pharmacy.

Fragrances Little to no perfume (or other fragrance) is recommended when working behind a pharmacy counter, and may extend to other fragrances, such as laundry detergent and shampoos. There are many people, both employees and patients, who are allergic to different fragrances. These reactions can range from mild irritation to difficulty breathing. As with food preparation, medication dispensing uses many of the same principles of cleanliness.

Wearing Pharmacy Identification

Name badges must always be worn while working in the pharmacy, not only so customers or patients can identify you as an employee, but so other employees can as well. In a hospital setting, there may be hundreds of employees. Your ID badge may be the only way you can access the facility and begin work. It is often used to clock into the payroll system and to unlock secured areas of a facility.

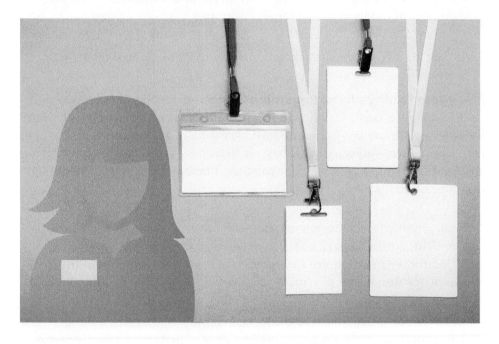

Know Your Facility's Policies Depending on the setting, your ID badge may look different. It could be simple with only your name and title on it, or it could include your photo, name, title, and department. Typically, only your first name will be listed, or your first name and the first initial of your last name. Limiting the personal information that can be gained on an ID badge helps to ensure your safety and security as an employee.

Recognize the Impact of Pharmacy Identification in the Workplace In other types of employment, forgetting your badge may be an acceptable error to make. Often there is a blank badge available to use on which you can fill in your name, or you just go through your day without one. In the pharmacy department, you may have to go back home to retrieve your ID if you forgot it because of its importance.

Practice Tip

It is a common mistake to forget your badge in the rush to get ready and go to work. One habit to employ can be to leave your badge in your car, such as in your glove box, so it always travels with you.

Patient/Customer Concerns One of the most important elements of healthcare safety in the pharmacy is accountability. Many unique scenarios come up each day that are handled by different technicians and pharmacists. When a patient or other healthcare practitioner follows up with the pharmacy team, knowing which person they originally worked with can save time and improve communication. Wearing proper identification helps improve customer care.

Pharmacy Security Issues Due to the street value of controlled substances, there is always a potential for theft or robbery of these medications from a pharmacy. Security precautions apply for all settings, including keypad or biometric locks on entrances and secure storage for CII medications. Your ID badge is one of these measures that keeps your workplace secure.

EXPAND YOUR KNOWLEDGE

Pharmacy Security

Many security measures are used, including employee identification, to secure a pharmacy. Cameras, panic alarms, as well as policies and procedures for specific events are all layers of security to keep employees and patients safe and medications secure. Even the design of most retail pharmacies is planned with security in mind. Placing a pharmacy towards the back of the store, increases the time a potential criminal must travel to reach the pharmacy, which also means a longer exit. This distance can discourage potential criminals. For more information on security measures used in pharmacies, review this article from *U.S. Pharmacist*: https://SSPharm. ParadigmEducation.com/PharmacySecurity.

3.3 Body Language

Nonverbal communication provides an abundance of information but is often the aspect of communication and professionalism that we think about the least. When it comes to professional image, how confident we appear is often indicated not only by what we say but also by how we walk, gesture with our hands, smile, make eye contact, or how we shake someone's hand.

> **"The impressions gained by these actions can have a profound impact on the perception that patients have of the pharmacy and affect the trust they place in our care."**

The impressions gained by these actions can have a profound impact on the perception that patients have of the pharmacy and affect the trust they place in our care.

The concept of body language and its use is further developed in another chapter, but its connection to professional image and how you present to patients and other healthcare providers must be included here. Because this is typically an unconscious element of our behavior, there can never be too much time dedicated to its development.

Checking Your Body Language

If a person can tell you are having a bad day just by looking at you, you should consider adjusting your body language. Consider your own facial expressions, gestures, and posture and how they might be interpreted (or misinterpreted) by others.

Consider Facial Expression When a patient comes to fill a prescription, there are expectations that must be met for the patient to continue to do business at your facility. The patient expects that the staff will be friendly, caring, and competent. Facial expressions go a long way to conveying that impression. A warm smile, eye contact, and sympathetic expressions let the patient know you want to help the patient get better and that you care about the patient's personal circumstances.

Note Hand and Arm Gestures Using your hands to help tell a story or describe what you are talking about is a very common trait and useful for telling a great story or making a point. In a professional setting, however, excessive use of hand and arm gestures can be seen as manic or *too* excited, which can affect the impression of the pharmacy in general. Keep gestures subdued, and use them only when necessary to convey a message.

Also consider how you are holding your arms. Crossing your arms across your body can be misinterpreted as a display of boredom or aggression, even if the person doing so is simply cold.

Correct Your Posture Walking, standing, and sitting with an upright position projects confidence. It makes you look more capable, and it can give you a greater sense of poise and confidence. Practice using correct posture in sitting, standing, and walking. For an upright stance, balance your weight on both feet, and center your core body weight between them. See Figure 3.1.

Figure 3.1 Proper Standing Posture

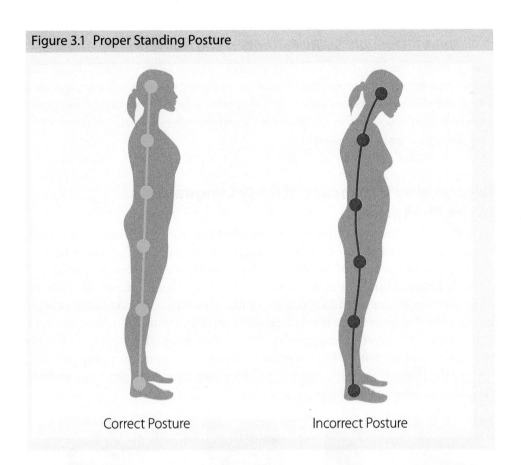

Correct Posture   Incorrect Posture

Sitting up straight means holding up your head, relaxing your shoulders down and slightly back, aligning your spine perpendicular to your thighs, and putting your feet flat on the floor. Your balance should be centered over both of your hips, with your chin straight out. See Figure 3.2.

Figure 3.2 Proper Sitting Posture

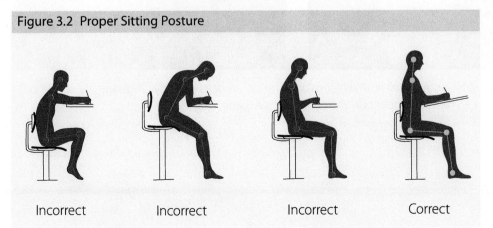

Incorrect   Incorrect   Incorrect   Correct

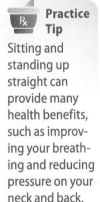

Practice Tip

Sitting and standing up straight can provide many health benefits, such as improving your breathing and reducing pressure on your neck and back.

Recognizing the Impact of Body Language in the Workplace

As with coworkers and supervisors, nonverbal gestures, expressions, or movements can help or hinder communications with customers. If you aren't careful, you can communicate exactly the opposite message you intended by body language alone. For example, working on a computer while talking with a patient might seem like you are being very efficient and multitasking, but the fact that your body is still facing the terminal while you are glancing at the patient will give the impression that you do not really want to talk with the patient and are not giving the patient enough attention. Stopping, turning toward the person, and fully listening will convey care and a desire to address the patient's concern properly.

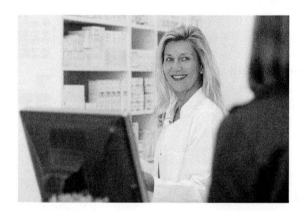 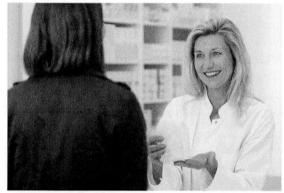

Which stance is more welcoming? The differences in body language are subtle but can have an impact on the customer's experience.

3.4 Module Summary

All the aspects of professional appearance discussed in this module have a profound impact on your potential career path as a pharmacy technician. Attention spent on your appearance and professional image create an overall impression to supervisors of your capacity to work with or manage others. You may be a stellar pharmacy technician, but if hygiene is an issue, you will not be a good fit with the rest of the department. Projecting a proper professional image and adjusting to professional expectations lets your supervisor and managers know that you can handle advanced roles and interactions.

Many elements of your appearance and hygiene will be noticed within seconds in a workplace. By knowing proper grooming and clothing standards for the pharmacy, you will be best able to present a professional image. This knowledge will help you to not only secure employment in any given pharmacy setting, but also will allow you to interact with colleagues and patients in a more professional manner. These elements can help with advancement in your own career and have the added benefit of elevating the profession as a whole.

These elements of professional image take time to cultivate. Habits in personal hygiene and appearance do not change overnight. Effort and attention must be spent on these different aspects to develop mastery. Support this mastery by treating your classes like the workplace. Follow the dress code daily. Always wear your ID badge. Practice standing and sitting with good posture, and be mindful of your facial expressions and gestures. The effort in all these areas create an effective professional presence that will take you a long way on your career journey.

 The online course includes additional review and assessment resources.

Professional Behavior

LEARNING OBJECTIVES

1 Develop a personal professional image. (Section 4.1)

2 Understand professional behaviors that lead to success. (Section 4.2)

3 Demonstrate professional behaviors. (Section 4.2)

4 Understand professional courtesies. (Section 4.3)

5 Learn how to manage interpersonal interactions professionally. (Section 4.4)

6 Understand codes of conduct and company culture. (Section 4.5)

To view the *ASHP/ACPE Accreditation Standards* addressed in this chapter, refer to Appendix A.

The way you behave on the job conveys the level of importance you place on your career. Just as you learned in Module 3, first impressions matter, and your professional behavior shapes how employers, colleagues, and customers view you.

In this module, you will review the importance of maintaining a professional image, applying common professional behaviors and etiquette rules, fostering good interpersonal professional behaviors, and following company standards regarding professional behavior.

4.1 Professional Image and Behavior

Recall that professional image describes the way an individual presents themselves in relation to their profession. **Professional image** is the combination of traits, such as professional actions, competence, poise, attire, and credibility. These traits together illustrate your professionalism. **Professional behaviors** are the actions you take in the workplace that demonstrate your ability to solve problems; act ethically; remain calm under pressure; and treat colleagues, supervisors, and customers politely and with respect.

Work Wise

Your reputation speaks for itself. Demonstrate your professionalism—show, don't tell.

Your actions can affect your professional image. If you are not efficient with your time in the pharmacy, colleagues have to compensate, causing them to think poorly of you as a professional. Professional image directly affects your **professional reputation**, the beliefs or opinions that others have about your performance in the workplace. If people believe you are trustworthy and reliable, they are more likely to give you important tasks and responsibilities. Supervisors will know your reputation as someone who can be relied upon, which can lead to promotions over time.

Transitioning from Student to Pharmacy Professional

A student's behavior includes actions, such as going to class on time, studying for tests, and working well with other students on group projects. Most of these actions are good training for the workplace. However, the stakes are higher as you transition from a student to a pharmacy professional. Making a mistake in a lab course won't have the potentially life-threatening results that making a mistake in a compounding facility will. Being a student is the best time to cultivate professional behavior while you are still learning and can afford to make mistakes.

The same behaviors that make you successful in the academic environment translate to the workplace. For example, if you successfully fulfill your part of a team presentation, you are likely to get a higher grade as well as gain the trust and respect of your classmates; completing your assigned duties in the pharmacy can positively affect your performance review, promote company goals, and improve relationships with your colleagues. Punctuality, dedication, and attention to detail are among the skills honed in the academic setting. If you were not highly successful in certain areas, such as attendance, understand that you must correct these to succeed in the field.

Employers are looking for certain traits in their new hires that go beyond academic competencies and specialized skills. In his 2012 report *Planning Your School-to-Career Transition*, John J. Liptak, EdD, said that many employers complain that while new employees brought many technical skills to the workplace, they often lacked the skills to manage their careers and be effective employees. The skills new employees lacked included successfully adapting to the workplace, managing stress, and navigating workplace relationships.

A classroom and lab setting can be very controlled and structured. These environments teach the technical skills needed to be a competent technician. However, be ready to operate in a potentially chaotic and less-controlled setting in the workplace.

EXPAND YOUR KNOWLEDGE

Views of Professionalism

In 2013, York College of Pennsylvania's Center for Professional Excellence asked 400 employers to complete its National Professionalism Survey. Nearly half of the respondents stated that less than 50% of college graduates displayed professionalism in their first year. In 2015, the center conducted a similar professionalism study among 519 recent college graduates. In that survey, 62.2% of respondents stated that they possessed the professionalism skills needed to succeed in a workplace. This discrepancy suggests that students feel as if they are well equipped with professional skills for the workplace, but employers see otherwise.

Learn from Experience The transition from student to pharmacy professional begins with your externship experience, continues through your job search and interviews, and must be sustained throughout your employment.

Any jobs you have held, even ones that do not directly relate to your career as a pharmacy technician, provided you with experiences in professional behavior. You have learned from your own interactions by observing others who demonstrate professional behavior and by making your own mistakes. Learning from experience is often referred to as *learned behavior*. Shadowing other technicians during an externship and learning how they communicate with customers will give you experiences to draw from when you are in the workplace.

In addition to learning from experience, you may want to seek guidance on workplace behavior from professional workshops and seminars, your hiring facility's handbook, and your own research.

Work Wise

Learn from other people's failures as much as their successes. By observing how *not* to do something, you can avoid making the same mistakes.

Cultivate Professional Behaviors The professional behaviors to cultivate as you make the transition from student to professional are being adaptable, managing stress, and navigating relationships. For example, when you are a student, you must adapt to your instructors' many different personality types. Some may be more personable, while others are strictly business with interactions. These experiences can apply to your first pharmacy position or externship. You will learn to identify and adapt to the personalities and work styles of your supervisors and switch your style to match.

Another important behavior you will learn as a student and translate to the workplace is successfully managing stress. When you are a student, you encounter many stressors, such as managing competing deadlines, difficult assignments, difficult classmates, and your personal life and coursework. As a professional, you have to manage multiple prescriptions that all need to be filled, deal with difficult patients or coworkers, and manage work–life balance. Adapt the lessons you have learned as a student, and you will be more successful in the workplace.

> "The professional behaviors to cultivate as you make the transition from student to professional are being adaptable, managing stress, and navigating relationships."

These behaviors and other professional behaviors will be covered in more detail throughout this module.

Creating a Professional Image through Behavior

Once you have gained a position or been placed in an externship, you will begin to cultivate a professional image. As described previously, you will use the experiences you have gained as a student and in your externship to guide how to behave in the field. These behaviors have a direct effect on how your colleagues view you and consequently on your overall success in your new career.

To create a professional image, consider how you currently view yourself.

Recognize the Effect of Self-Perception One of the most important factors of behavior is how you perceive yourself, known as **self-perception**. Your behavior reveals your temperament, self-confidence, and self-esteem.

Your temperament, mood, and emotions play a large part in your behavior. **Temperament** is defined as the combination of a person's mental, physical, and emotional traits and natural disposition. It is considered innate and cannot be changed. There are many different temperaments—some people may be naturally outgoing and active, while others are quieter and more cautious. Knowing your temperament can help you learn how to develop effective professional behaviors that align with it. For example, if you are a shy person, you may need extra practice to work up the courage to serve customers at a pharmacy, or you might choose a role that does not require such interactions.

Personality is another important aspect to behavior. **Personality** is defined as the collection of thoughts, feelings, and behaviors that are associated with a person. Personality is different from temperament, because it is considered more malleable and is acquired on top of temperament. Personality is affected by factors such as education, culture, and experiences.

Your personality and temperament have an effect on how you behave, both in and out of the workplace. Understanding your natural and learned behaviors will help you determine what areas you might need to focus on while developing a professional image.

EXPAND YOUR KNOWLEDGE

The Four Tendencies

Gretchen Rubin, author of the book *The Four Tendencies*, says there are four personality types that affect how people respond to internal and external expectations: obligers, upholders, questioners, and rebels. Obligers respond best to external expectations. For example, they will straighten the pharmacy shelves because their supervisor asked them to, though if not specifically asked, obligers probably would not complete the task. Upholders are both internally and externally motivated. If they think the shelves need to be organized, they will do so of their own volition.

Questioners need workplace tasks to make sense. If a supervisor asks them to do something, they want to know why it is important. Rebels will struggle to do a task if they do not want to. They may decide they would rather file the faxed prescriptions than attend to the shelves.

Knowing what personality type you align with and how it relates to your motivation in the workplace can be a very useful tool. To learn more, read the article "How the Four Tendencies Changed Our Workplace" at **https://SSPharm .ParadigmEducation.com/FourTendencies**.

Other important factors in your self-perception are self-confidence and self-esteem. People who are **self-confident** trust their abilities, qualities, and judgments. Someone who is self-confident is able to recognize when a prescription has a potential error and feels confident in bringing it to the pharmacist's attention. People who are self-confident often have high self-esteem. **Self-esteem** is having intrinsic belief in one's own worth as a person.

To measure your own self-confidence and self-esteem, complete the following Self-Reflection. Once you have determined your level of self-confidence and self-esteem, you will see how they relate to your behaviors in the workplace. An honest evaluation of your self-esteem allows you to identify areas of strength and of weakness. By building on your strengths and being aware of weaknesses, you will greatly increase your confidence and self-worth, making you a much more effective technician.

Self-Reflection:
How High Are Your Self-Esteem and Confidence?

For each of the statements, answer "always," "sometimes," or "rarely/never." Respond to statements as honestly as possible.

Self-Esteem Statements	Always	Sometimes	Rarely/Never
I get upset if someone criticizes me, even if it is constructive.			
I usually ask other people what they think I should do before deciding on a course of action.			
I feel uncomfortable when someone compliments me.			
I find myself apologizing for things often, even if I'm not really at fault.			
I think that overall, people find me boring to talk to.			
I feel that I will never amount to anything significant.			
I feel people will respect me only if I'm good looking and/or successful.			
I feel I will never be as skilled or as smart as I should be.			
I am not confident I've done a good job unless someone else points it out.			
I avoid having arguments with others because I don't want them to get angry or dislike me.			
Subtotal per column	_____ x5	_____ x3	_____ x1

Tally Your Score: Always = 5 points; Sometimes = 3 points; Rarely/Never = 1 point

Total Score: _____

40 to 50 points: This score indicates you have high self-esteem and confidence and a positive self-image.

25 to 39 points: This score indicates you are aware of some personal strengths but also dwell on negative aspects. More work can be done to increase your self-perception.

Below 25 points: This score indicates a need for immediate attention on your self-esteem. While there are always areas to work on, there are many positive elements that you already possess and need to identify.

Your results from this self-evaluation are a good indication of how others perceive your confidence and competence. You should take these results seriously and consider following the advice for improving your self-image.

Create a Positive Social Perception Your professional image is shaped not only by how you think of yourself but also by others' perceptions of you. Your behavior determines if your supervisors, colleagues, and customers view you as trustworthy, motivated, flexible, and hard-working. If you create a positive social perception, others will want to work with you, and supervisors will want to hire you.

Sometimes, there can be a discrepancy between how you see yourself and how others view you. For example, you may see yourself as confident and outgoing, but your colleagues may view the same behavior as cocky and obnoxious.

To create a positive social perception and eliminate any discrepancies, observe others' reactions, ask for feedback, and make improvements.

Observation During workplace interactions, observe how your colleagues react to you. If you bring up an error, are they defensive? Do they avoid having friendly, personal conversations with you? You may be inadvertently making people uncomfortable by being too abrasive or talkative.

Feedback Ask your supervisor for feedback to determine your social perception in the workplace. When you know your strengths and weaknesses, you can begin to improve your behavior.

Improvements After you have determined how others view you, make improvements to your behavior to ensure that you have a positive social perception.

Understand the Effect of Professional Behavior on Career Success
Professional behavior affects your career trajectory. If you exhibit poor professional behavior on a regular basis, you will have a harder time getting promoted or being considered for other opportunities. Tardiness or rudeness to customers will lead to disciplinary action. Maintaining professional relationships is also extremely important when looking for other career opportunities. If your colleagues think highly of you, they are more likely to recommend you as a candidate when you are searching for a new position.

Recognizing the Effect of Professional Behavior on the Workplace

While it is easy to see that your behavior has a major effect on the trajectory of your career, you might not realize that it also influences many areas in the workplace. For example, your behavior directly affects workflow. In a retail pharmacy, if you are late or procrastinating, having personal conversations, or wasting time, prescriptions are not getting filled. This backup results in angry customers and can also disrupt other tasks that need to be completed.

Your behavior also affects workplace culture. **Workplace culture** includes employee morale, job satisfaction, and camaraderie. If you have a negative

 Work Wise

Just because you think something is true doesn't mean it is. Be conscious of others' reactions to you and your behavior for an accurate assessment.

attitude at work or complain about other employees, supervisors, or the company at large, you are bringing down the morale of your colleagues. If you are always gossiping with colleagues, for example, you will not be seen as trustworthy, and your coworkers may avoid talking to and confiding in you.

Your workplace has a public image as well, and its employees are a direct reflection of the company. You have to behave professionally not only at work but also outside of work to help the company maintain a professional image.

> ### Think It Through: Social Media and Professionalism
> How does your social media profile reflect on you professionally? Would you want a supervisor or person in your workplace to see your posts or photos? How could you cultivate a more professional online image?

4.2 Professional Workplace Behaviors

One of the most valued professional behaviors is having a good work ethic. **Work ethic** is the principle that hard work is virtuous and worthy of reward. In a recent study on career readiness conducted by the National Association of Colleges and Employers, those who hire college graduates were asked which professional competencies were essential to workplace success. Professionalism/work ethic topped the list with 97.5% of respondents identifying it as either "absolutely essential" or "essential" for a new college hire's success.

Work ethic is driven by both intrinsic values (such as the satisfaction that comes from doing good work and helping others) and extrinsic values (such as job recognition and job security). Work ethic is also shaped by many factors, including positive attitude, initiative/motivation, and dependability.

Additionally, good etiquette and professional courtesies are important elements of professional workplace behavior.

Identifying Desired Personal Behaviors

In 2014, CareerBuilder conducted a national online survey of 2,138 hiring managers and human resource professionals to gauge the importance of soft skills in the workplace. The majority (77%) reported that soft skills are as important as hard skills (job–specific skills or competencies) when reviewing a potential job candidate. In fact, 16% of respondents said that soft skills are *more important* than hard skills. Some of the most desired soft skills are illustrated in Figure 4.1.

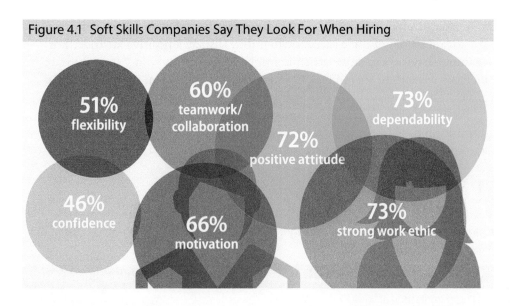

Figure 4.1 Soft Skills Companies Say They Look For When Hiring

51% flexibility

60% teamwork/collaboration

72% positive attitude

73% dependability

46% confidence

66% motivation

73% strong work ethic

Some of the desired personal behaviors and traits to cultivate as a pharmacy technician are a positive attitude, initiative, self-direction, competency in pharmacy skills, focus, honesty, integrity, flexibility, dependability, accountability, leadership, emotional intelligence, and critical-thinking skills.

Adopt a Positive Attitude **Attitude** is a way of thinking or feeling about someone or something, and it affects an individual's actions or behaviors. Attitude also dictates how a person responds to stressful situations. In the workplace, the effects of negative and positive thinking affect your colleagues, your job performance, and your career success, as shown in Figure 4.2.

Figure 4.2 Effects of Negative and Positive Thinking

Effects of Negative Thinking	Effects of Positive Thinking
Undermines relationships with coworkers and workplace climate and culture	Feels happy and passes this on to coworkers, improving workplace culture
Feels less engaged and is less productive	Feels more engaged and is more productive
Feels victimized, does not get perks or additional responsibilities	Is cooperative, grateful, and trusted, does get perks and responsibilities
Is less likely to advance and more likely to leave	Is more likely to stay and advance
Risks job security and is more likely to be laid off	Feels less stress and is more secure in job
Experiences less confidence and low performance or achievements, individually and on teams	Feels more confident, creative, and empowered to achieve, individually and on teams
Experiences identification problem	Feels more grounded in career
Offers poor customer service and is a bad reflection on business to public	Provides better customer service and is a good reflection on business to public

Leaders in many industries, including pharmacy, recognize the effects on the advancement of their careers when they display a positive attitude. For example, having a positive attitude might help impress your externship site mentors enough to stay in touch with you—and keep you in mind when a position becomes available.

Positive thinking can be automatic. However, some people have a predisposition toward negativity. To assess your positivity or negativity in the workplace, complete the following Self-Reflection.

 Self-Reflection:
How Positive Are You?

For each of the statements, answer "always," "sometimes," or "rarely/never." Respond to statements as honestly as possible.

When I am at work, I...	Always	Sometimes	Rarely/Never
speak in a friendly tone of voice.			
smile and use people's names while speaking with them.			
show a genuine interest in others.			
strive to do the best work possible.			
treat others with patience and tolerance.			
praise others generously.			
ask questions and listen openly to their responses.			
consider others' feelings and points of view.			
communicate openly and honestly.			
can be counted on to do the right thing.			
solve problems instead of complaining.			
support others in decision-making processes.			
take a win-win approach to resolving conflict.			
work well as part of a team.			
have a good sense of humor.			
stay committed to reaching organizational goals.			
focus on the process as well as the results.			
take responsibility for the quality of my work.			
demonstrate personal motivation.			
maintain a proactive attitude.			
Subtotal per column	_____ x5	_____ x3	_____ x1

Continues...

Tally Your Score: Always = 5 points; Sometimes = 3 points; Rarely/Never = 1 point

Total Score: _____

80 to 100 points: This score indicates you have a strong foundation for having a positive attitude at work.

50 to 79 points: This score indicates that although you are positive at work some of the time, you should work on increasing your positivity on a more consistent basis.

Below 50 points: This score indicates a need for attention to develop a more positive attitude and deeper commitment to the overall success of the organization.

Show Initiative and Self-Direction Taking initiative is important in the workplace. That initiative might include volunteering to fill in for a colleague, thinking of new ways to accomplish tasks, doing tasks that nobody else wants to or has time for, or staying late to complete a project. For example, if you have an idea of a better way to complete a cart-fill order, you may draft a proposal and create a document that shows how technicians will use your new system. This shows initiative and creativity and can help you get noticed in the workplace.

Self-direction is also a quality that employers want in their employees. You need to be able to work on an assigned task with minimal oversight, set deadlines for yourself, and solve problems on your own. If you are having a conflict with another technician, it is important to attempt to solve the problem on your own before going to the pharmacist. Being proactive about problems will help you maintain a professional image and allow the pharmacist to focus on more important tasks.

Demonstrate Competencies Throughout your academic career as a pharmacy technician student, you have acquired important knowledge and skills. You will demonstrate this knowledge not only on a résumé and during your job search but also within your career once you are in the field. Employers look to build teams that draw from a variety of skill sets and work well together. If you excel at extemporaneous compounding and math, demonstrate it to your employer to make it clear you can be relied upon for these activities. Being the go-to person for a particular task is invaluable to a pharmacy.

Maintain a Work Focus As you learned in Module 1, an important aspect of being successful in your career is managing time well. Working hard to complete your daily, weekly, and monthly goals demonstrates that you take your career seriously.

It is hard to achieve your professional goals and maintain a professional image if you are constantly distracted. Avoid unprofessional behaviors, such as making personal phone calls, sending text messages, surfing the internet,

Practice Tip

The company you work for should have values and policies that promote honesty and integrity. If your company is not as ethical as it should be, consider searching for an employer with values that align with yours.

and spreading gossip, all of which can serve as major distractions to getting your tasks done during the workday.

Act with Honesty and Integrity **Honesty** is the fairness and straight-forwardness of your conduct as well as the adherence to facts. **Integrity** refers to one's adherence to a code of moral values. These two qualities are linked together—acting with honesty means being truthful and straightforward, while acting with integrity means adhering to moral principles. One can be honest while not having integrity, but one cannot have integrity without being honest. These traits are both important behaviors to consistently exhibit in the workplace. Below are some examples of how you can demonstrate integrity in your career:

- Present yourself honestly in your résumé, cover letter, and letters of reference.
- Adhere to your facility's policies and procedures.
- Do not use equipment, such as computers and phones, for personal use.
- Never steal supplies (or medications) from the workplace.
- Don't accept praise for someone else's work.

Show Flexibility Pharmacy practice is always changing. New technologies mean that workflow and responsibilities will shift, such as when pharmacies began to accept escripts in addition to paper prescriptions. The roles of a pharmacy technician are shifting as well. As more pharmacists take on patient counseling and care, pharmacy technicians take on greater responsibilities, such as tech-check-tech, medication reconciliation, and medication therapy management. These changes are not consistent across all states, but employers are still seeking technicians that can adapt to the changing field.

Flexibility is defined as the willingness to change or compromise. Being willing to change work responsibilities, priorities, expectations, and environments shows that you are flexible. Flexibility may also mean going outside your job description or regular work hours to accomplish tasks.

> ### Think It Through: Learning New Skills
> Many healthcare employees are resistant to change. Have you ever had to learn a new skill set or be trained on new technology in the workplace? How did you respond?

Demonstrate Dependability and Accountability **Dependability** is the quality of being able to be relied upon. If your supervisors see you as someone who they can count on, you are more likely to get positive performance reviews, challenging projects, and promotions. Consider an employee who always meets deadlines, double-checks work, and rarely makes mistakes. Now consider someone who often misses deadlines and does sloppy work. Who is more likely to be a lead technician or supervisor?

Even the most careful and diligent employees make mistakes, however. **Accountability** is taking responsibility for one's actions. If you make a mistake, it is important to admit where you went wrong, identify an acceptable solution, and learn from the mistake. For example, if you mixed up two soundalike drugs on the shelves, it is important to quickly rectify the situation and place the items in their proper places. Instead of blaming an external factor—"I was distracted by all the customers waiting in line"—it is important to be accountable and say, "I made a mistake. I was placing items on the shelves while trying to serve customers and got distracted." Accountability is discussed more in depth in Module 5.

Display Leadership Because you will be starting out in an entry-level position, you may not consider the importance of leadership early in your career. However, you do not need to *be* in a leadership position to *act* like a leader. The following are common qualities of a leader:

- organized
- confident
- fair
- respectful
- influential

> "You do not need to *be* in a leadership position to *act* like a leader."

To show you are leadership minded, do not be afraid to go above and beyond your assigned responsibilities. Volunteering to take on extra work shows that you are interested in advancing in your career and willing to do what it takes to achieve your goals. If there are opportunities to work in teams, you can assume a leadership role and demonstrate how you are organized, confident, and fair with your team. Once you have some experience in your job, offer to help newer employees learn their roles and responsibilities. This training offers you the opportunity to display leadership to your supervisors, can help strengthen your own skills, and help build camaraderie with teammates.

Demonstrate Emotional Intelligence **Emotional intelligence** is the ability to control your emotions and identify the emotions of others around you. When we think of intelligence, we often think of it in the classical sense: people who are intelligent are "book smart" and have a depth of knowledge on specific subjects. However, employers say that they are looking for employees with high levels of emotional intelligence, not necessarily employees who are classically intelligent.

According to Daniel Goleman, psychologist and author of *Emotional Intelligence*, 67% of all abilities associated with a strong job performance are related to emotional intelligence. Goleman, the first to apply the concept of emotional intelligence to business, listed five elements of emotional intelligence:

- self-awareness
- self-regulation
- motivation
- empathy
- social skills

"67% of all abilities associated with a strong job performance are related to emotional intelligence."

Self-Awareness Emotionally intelligent employees know their strengths and weaknesses. If you struggle with a particular type of calculation, you should not pretend to know how to do it and risk making a dangerous mistake. Instead, you should admit to your colleagues that you struggle with certain calculations and ask them for help. Emotionally intelligent employees are also open to learning how to improve their weaknesses.

Self-Regulation **Self-regulation** is being able to control one's emotions. When dealing with difficult customers, emotionally intelligent people have developed ways of coping. For example, they might know that they need to take five deep breaths before responding to a demanding customer.

Motivation Emotionally intelligent workers are also motivated. They consistently work toward their goals and maintain a high work ethic. They take pride in the work they produce.

Empathy Empathy is the ability to understand and share the feelings of others. Empathy is an extremely important quality to have as a pharmacy technician. There will be many times in your career when you encounter patients dealing with major life struggles—such as a parent whose child is going through cancer treatments or customers who just lost their jobs and are struggling to pay for medications. If you can put yourself in those patients' shoes, you will be able to provide them with respectful, courteous, and empathetic care.

Social Skills People with good social skills act as team players, helping to strengthen the entire department. There are often many different personalities among pharmacists and technicians working together. Social skills can help resolve difficult interpersonal problems. The techniques of effective communication are covered in Module 5.

Engage in Critical Thinking and Problem Solving **Critical thinking** is the objective analysis and evaluation of an issue to form a judgment. In the workplace, you may rely upon the objective information you learned in school (i.e., knowing which drugs have which side effects, how to dose medications, etc.), but more often, you will be challenged with critical-thinking problems to solve. For example, what do you do when you are filling an order for 10 pills and have exactly 10 in stock, and then you drop one on the floor? Or how would you handle a situation in which you have three patients waiting for the same inhaler drug but only two inhaler drugs are on the shelf? How would you choose which patients to serve and which to keep waiting? Learning how to develop critical-thinking skills is an important part of developing a professional image. Critical thinking and problem solving are covered more in depth in Module 2.

EXPAND YOUR KNOWLEDGE

Importance of Critical Thinking

In 2012, the Chronicle of Higher Education and American Public Media's *Marketplace* conducted a survey among employers to understand their perceptions of the role of colleges in career preparation. This survey, titled *The Role of Higher Education in Career Development: Employer* *Perceptions*, focused on the discrepancies between the soft skills new hires possessed and the soft skills needed by employers in different industries. In the healthcare field, the largest discrepancy occurred in the survey area of making decisions and problem solving.

4.3 Professional Courtesies

Courtesy is defined as behaviors that display manners and respect for others. Showing courtesy in a pharmacy leads to satisfied patients and potentially advances your career as a technician. These courtesies apply both to customers and coworkers.

Self-Reflection:
Consider Your Professional Courtesies

For each of the statements, answer "always," "sometimes," or "rarely/never." Respond to statements as honestly as possible.

When interacting with coworkers and customers, I...	Always	Sometimes	Rarely/Never
say good morning, afternoon, or evening.			
say please and thank you.			
clean up after myself.			
am attentive during staff meetings.			
am courteous in phone interactions.			
am mindful of noise level while speaking.			

Continues...

When interacting with coworkers and customers, I...	Always	Sometimes	Rarely/Never
am respectful of coworker privacy and space.			
stay home when contagious with illness.			
hold doors or elevators for people.			
keep my professional and personal life separate.			
Subtotal per column	_____ x5	_____ x3	_____ x1

Tally Your Score: Always = 5 points; Sometimes = 3 points; Rarely/Never = 1 point

Total Score: _____

41 to 50 points: You have excellent professional presence.

31 to 40 points: Your current level of professional presence is satisfactory; however, there is room for improvement.

Below 30 points: You have poor professional presence, and you should work quickly and diligently to improve your skills.

Greeting Someone Appropriately

Your first chance to display your professional presence occurs when you meet your potential preceptor or employer. Good eye contact, a firm handshake, and professional introduction convey confidence and competence. Make a habit of initiating a professional greeting when you meet someone in both personal and professional situations. This will help you gain confidence for times when the greeting truly matters, such as a job interview. Here are some principles to apply when greeting someone appropriately for the first time:

- Stand when you are introduced to someone.
- Give your full name and say it clearly and not too fast.
- Listen carefully to the person's name and use it in the initial conversation to remember it. Use a person's formal title when addressing them until told differently.

There are three types of formal introductions for which you should prepare: meeting someone you don't know (in which you initiate the introduction), meeting someone who has been introduced to you, and meeting a person of influence (i.e., potential employer, supervisor, business owner, etc.).

Introduce Yourself When meeting people for the first time, always state your name and use an appropriate greeting. Wait for others to give their name, or if necessary, politely ask for their name so that you can engage in a discussion. For example, you might say, "Hello, I wanted to introduce myself.

My name is Sarah Martinez; it's very nice to meet you." If they forget to state their name, you can follow with, "I'm sorry, I did not catch your name."

The key is to then swiftly switch your brain over to "listening mode" so that you can pay attention to the other person's name. Many people don't remember it even after hearing it because of the stress of meeting someone new. Reply right away, using the person's name. Saying the name aloud will help you remember it. For example, you might say, "Great to meet you, Jamal. Are you here for the conference today?" When being introduced to someone new by way of a third party (e.g., a coworker who is introducing you to another coworker), use the other person's name first and then give your name. For example, this type of exchange may sound something like, "Sarah, this is Jamal. You'll be working with him a lot."

Introduce Yourself to Leaders When you are meeting a leader (e.g., pharmacist, manager, company owner, CEO, or direct supervisor) for the first time in person, you might say, "Hello, Mr. Jackson. My name is Sarah. We spoke on the phone last week to set up the interview. It's nice to meet you in person." Lastly, if meeting your supervising pharmacist for the first time, you might say, "Hello, Ms. Andrews. I'm Sarah. It is a pleasure to meet you. I am really looking forward to working for you."

Projecting Confidence and Respect in a Handshake

In most introductions, it is appropriate and important to shake the hand of the person you are meeting. A weak handshake gives a poor impression; one that is too strong projects domination or a challenge—a clear lack of understanding of basic etiquette. Figure 4.3 illustrates different types of handshakes. As you extend your hand, follow these important principles:

- Smile and make eye contact.
- Always shake hands using your right hand. (If you are holding something with your right hand, set the item down.)
- Make sure your handshake is firm but not crushing.
- Shake hands using an up-and-down motion.
- Be aware that a handshake should be between three and five seconds in duration.
- Shake the entire hand and not just the other person's fingers.
- Do not pat or place your left hand on top of the other person's hand unless it is a particularly friendly and personal situation.
- If your palms are sweaty, subtly wipe your palm on the side of your hip before shaking hands.

Figure 4.3 Types of Handshakes

The traditional handshake occurs when the right hands of each person are firmly interlocked in a side-by-side manner, and the shake goes up and down.

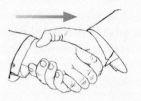 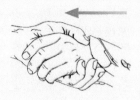 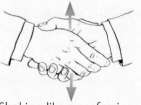

| Taking control | Giving control | Shaking like a professional |

© Czaroot, Dreamstime.com

 WORKPLACE WISDOM

Don't Be Patient Zero

If you are feeling as though you might be coming down with a cold or the flu, wash your hands thoroughly before being introduced to others, and do not touch your face. You don't want to be patient zero and cause an outbreak. If you are obviously sick, politely decline the person's handshake and say, "I'm sorry. I'd rather not shake your hand; I've been under the weather and don't want to risk making you sick." Then express what a pleasure it is to meet the person.

Practicing Everyday Courtesies and Manners

The first and foremost key to professional courtesy is to always say "please" and "thank you." Other common courtesies to use in your professional life include turning off your phone at work; listening carefully to others; paying for your portion for any shared expenses, such as group lunches; and respecting people's time off by not contacting them about work issues after work hours (unless it is an emergency).

Other important ways to display good manners include the following:

- Do not use profanity.
- Do not discuss personal issues at work, especially in front of patients.
- Ask about how others are doing, but do not brag or talk only about yourself.
- Avoid talking loudly on your cell phone or using the speakerphone function.
- Do not check your phone or text while talking to someone.

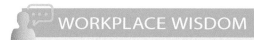
Remember Breakroom Etiquette

You must continue to act professionally even while on a break. Observe these basic manners and courtesies regarding the lunch/break room and while dining with others:

- Eat only food that you have brought.

- Do not use too much space in the refrigerator or leave food in there for multiple days.

- If you take the last of the coffee, start a new pot.

- Do not cook food with strong odors.

- If there are shared foods or treats, take only one.

- Clean up after yourself by wiping off counters and throwing away your garbage.

- Do not leave dishes in the sink or food in the drain.

4.4 Interpersonal Workplace Behaviors

Employers desire certain interpersonal behaviors in their employees. **Interpersonal** relates to relationships and communication between people. Having relationships that function well in a workplace helps productivity, job satisfaction, and overall goals. Any time there are many people of different backgrounds and different personalities all working together on a team, there are likely to be some conflicts. However, cultivating certain desired interpersonal behaviors among all teammates will allow for good working relationships and teamwork.

By knowing that Miguel is not agreeable until he has his morning coffee or that Susan loves talking about her rescue animals volunteer work, you are able to socially interact with them to allow for a smoother workday. This ties to emotional intelligence discussed earlier and a general awareness of the dynamics between different personalities.

Identifying Desired Interpersonal Behaviors

Some of the interpersonal behaviors that employers hope their employees exhibit are respect, kindness, and trust. To lead a successful team, they also hope that their employees work together effectively on a team as well as manage conflict.

Show Respect and Kindness There are many common courtesies that help build strong teams and pleasant interpersonal relationships. Many of these courtesies do not directly relate to the work being done in the pharmacy but still help to build a strong workplace. Some ways to show respect and kindness include:

- using appropriate greetings
- showing interest in others' lives
- expressing empathy

Greeting colleagues appropriately when you come into work in the morning, for example, shows a level of kindness and respect. Another way to build strong relationships is to show interest in your colleague's lives. If you frequently forget their children's names or don't take an interest when they talk about their hobbies, you are demonstrating that you do not really care about your colleagues as people. But if you remember details and get to know people's interests outside of work, you are more likely to build and sustain a warm and respectful relationship.

Another way to show respect and kindness is to understand when others need a helping hand. Even if you are busy, if you offer to help coworkers put up inventory, they will consider you to be a team player. When a coworker is dealing with a frustrating customer, you can express empathy and offer solutions based on your own similar experiences.

Develop Trusting Relationships Trust is something that is built on consistent dependability. To develop a trusting relationship with your colleagues, you must follow through on your actions again and again. This consistency will help them see that you are someone of your word who will follow through with objectives. Having a strong commitment to the team is also important. If you are unwilling to go above and beyond, your relationships with your coworkers can suffer. For example, if your supervisor asks you to work extra shifts due to a staffing shortage, you are well within your rights to decline. But if you refuse, you will be letting down the rest of the team and causing others to have to take on more work.

Be an Effective Team Member As a student, you can probably point to some of the qualities you would like in a team member on a group project. You would want to work with someone who completes assigned tasks and is committed to getting the project done. The same can be said for a someone in the workplace. To be an effective team member, everyone needs to agree upon the roles and then carry out the tasks assigned to those roles. The team should aim for effective communication. Any conflicts should be addressed promptly, and everyone on the team should be accountable.

In a pharmacy that has delivery services, the entire team relies on each other to get the daily order out. The entry technician must generate the labels for delivery, and the filling tech needs to prepare the prescriptions in time for the delivery drivers to start their runs. The pharmacist must verify and make any counseling calls. If the team starts work at 6:00 a.m., and the pharmacy opens at 9:00 a.m., that's three hours to potentially prepare more than 100 orders for delivery. If one person on the team isn't contributing, everyone suffers.

Managing Conflict

How you manage conflict is a direct reflection of your professionalism. Employers want technicians who do their best to avoid conflict with others and who take proactive approaches to solving conflicts if they arise. Module 5 goes more in depth on ways to manage conflicts, but some basic strategies include the following:

- Communicate with the other person directly.
- Focus on behaviors, not personalities.
- Practice active listening skills (**active listening** is the act of fully listening to, concentrating on, and understanding what others say).
- Develop a plan to resolve the conflict with compromise.

For example, if another technician consistently does not mark opened stock bottles to indicate they are in use and have less than the full amount in them, it can cause problems with ordering. Instead of complaining about the technician to other coworkers (which is common), the strategies above can be used to manage the situation. Directly communicate with the technician, and ask about the unmarked bottles. Focus on the reason it is important instead of suggesting that the tech is lazy or forgetful. Listen to the reason for not completing the task. Ask if there is a way you can help resolve the situation. These strategies will allow for the problem to be addressed in a professional manner with less conflict than a passive-aggressive or other type of approach.

4.5 Company Standards of Behavior

Behavior is important to the success of your own career and also the company's. The way you and your coworkers behave on the job can affect the company's health. Unprofessional behavior can cost the company money—if you work slowly and procrastinate, certain goals will not be met. If you are terminated, the company must spend money on recruitment of and training for a replacement. To protect their businesses, most companies provide an employee handbook that helps identify appropriate behaviors, also known as a *code of conduct*. Companies also tend to have a more informal company culture, which helps guide appropriate staff behavior.

EXPAND YOUR KNOWLEDGE

A Code to Live By

A well-written code of conduct should leave no questions about how to operate in your place of business. An example would be CVS Pharmacy's code of conduct. It has guidelines on almost every potential interaction and behavior that you would encounter while working at the company. Items include accountability, how to talk to reporters or public officials, interpersonal relationships, leadership responsibilities, and more. These guidelines are effective in any retail setting and can give insight into what to expect for new technicians. The link to CVS's code of conduct can be found at **https://SSPharm.ParadigmEducation.com/CVSCode**.

Adhering to a Company's Code of Conduct

Every facility has a code of conduct that outlines the professional standards of behavior expected of its employees. If your behavior does not align with these standards, you risk losing your position at the company.

While every company is different, typical codes of conduct offer guidelines with regard to personal boundaries, romantic relationships, harassment, privacy, and safety (such as impairment and violence in the workplace).

Respect Personal and Professional Workplace Boundaries Having workplace boundaries is often expected in a company's code of conduct. While it is fine to be friendly with colleagues and to discuss your lives outside of the workplace, it can also be unprofessional if you do not know where the professional line is. For example, talking about how you tried a new restaurant over the weekend would be a good way to bond with coworkers, but talking about a night out drinking with friends would be unprofessional.

Spending time together outside of the workplace can be a difficult situation to navigate as well. Many coworkers like to spend time together, going to lunch or organizing a happy hour. Sometimes coworkers become good friends or even develop romantic interests. However, many companies have guidelines regarding romantic relationships.

Companies also have guidelines about different types of harassment and how to address them in the workplace.

Romantic Relationships It is not uncommon for coworkers to develop romantic feelings for one another. The key to professionally managing a romantic relationship in the workplace is to be very transparent. It might be tempting to keep it a secret, and it is good to practice discretion, but the best thing to do is to consult your company's code of conduct to see what the policies are for romantic relationships. Sometimes the rules indicate that relationships are acceptable, if they are disclosed and not between people of different power differentials (e.g., a relationship between a supervisor and direct report). Your company's human resources department can provide more information on how a romantic relationship is to be handled in your workplace.

Harassment **Discrimination** is when an employer is providing preferential treatment or mistreatment for reasons of age, gender, ethnicity, sexual orientation, religion, or other factors. Discrimination is illegal. **Harassment** is aggressive mistreatment, pressure, or intimidation that can be sexual or otherwise. These activities, particularly if they are of an ongoing or persistent nature, are not only unethical but also illegal.

If you find yourself the object of discrimination or harassment, first try to resolve the issue with the person or persons involved. Do your best to maintain your composure and to express your discomfort calmly and rationally. If possible, have a witness present to verify your communication. If discrimination or harassment persists, discuss the matter with a supervisor. The law requires all businesses, pharmacies included, to post information related to workplace discrimination and harassment.

> ### Think It Through: The Climate of Harassment
> With the rise of the #MeToo movement, there has been an increased spotlight on harassment and its effects in the workplace in many industries. Has there ever been a situation in which you or someone you knew experienced what would be considered harassment or discrimination? How did you or they handle it? If you haven't, how would you handle something like that if it occurred?

The US Equal Employment Opportunity Commission defines **sexual harassment** as "unwelcome sexual advances, requests for sexual favors, and other verbal or physical conduct of a sexual nature [that] constitutes sexual harassment when submission to or rejection of this conduct explicitly or implicitly affects an individual's employment, unreasonably interferes with an individual's work performance or creates an intimidating, hostile or offensive work environment." See Figure 4.4 for examples of harassment.

No one is allowed to create an unpleasant or uncomfortable work environment through sexual action, innuendo, or related means. Thus, you do not have to tolerate off-color or crude jokes if you do not wish to hear them. Nor can you contribute to creating an environment that is uncomfortable for your coworkers. One person's remark made in the spirit of fun can be the basis for another person's legal action.

If someone is offended by something you say or do, don't repeat the offense. If someone is doing something that bothers you, firmly say "stop." If the problem is not resolved by making yourself clear, follow up first with pharmacy management or the human resources department and then, if necessary, with upper-level management. If you are unsuccessful, as a last resort, make inquiries regarding the discrimination and harassment laws and procedures in your state.

Most community and hospital pharmacies have written policies and procedures to address such matters; follow the established protocol. If a facility's hiring or promotion practices fail to follow proper written procedures and guidelines, then the facility may be subject to a lawsuit.

Figure 4.4 Examples of Harassment

- inappropriate physical contact
- unwelcome sexual advances, requests for sexual favors, suggestive comments, inappropriate physical contact, and any other unwelcome verbal or physical conduct of a sexual nature
- displaying derogatory, vulgar, suggestive, or obscene pictures, cartoons, calendars, posters, or drawings
- threats or acts of violence and intimidation
- retaliation for reporting or threatening to report acts of misconduct or for reporting work-related injuries or illnesses

- comments, jokes, insults, slurs, offensive language, and other unwelcome actions that are offensive or stereotypical based upon age, religion, gender, sexual orientation, gender identity or expression, race, color, national origin, disability, military or veteran status, and any other protected category or personal characteristic

Recognize Workplace Safety Violations Workplace safety is of utmost importance when working in a pharmacy. Follow the safety guidelines outlined in your company's code of conduct. These rules and regulations will contribute to patient safety as well as employee and employer safety. Some common violations that are addressed in a code of conduct are guidelines relating to impairment and reckless or violent conduct.

Impairment Coming to work under the influence of alcohol or drugs can jeopardize the safety of patients, colleagues, and yourself. It can also lead to disciplinary action and, ultimately, termination.

While there are much greater restrictions and attention paid to narcotics in the pharmacy setting, the proximity to such potent chemicals is always a temptation to some. There are examples of technicians, pharmacists, nurses, and others who have become addicted to controlled substances or alcohol, which impaired their performance. In some cases, it has led to harm for a patient.

All state boards of pharmacy keep minutes of their meetings that are public record. Many contain specific examples of substance abuse and its effects on pharmacy operations.

If you have cause to suspect that a coworker is impaired, it is your ethical responsibility to report it for the safety of everyone in the department.

Reckless or Violent Conduct All company codes of conduct provide guidance regarding violent and reckless conduct in the workplace. Responding to a tense situation with violence shows a disregard for safety as well as demonstrates an inability to manage stress in the workplace. Reckless and violent conduct often leads to disciplinary action and/or termination.

Identifying Company Culture

Every company has its own unique **company culture** which is made up the following:

- values
- beliefs
- attitudes
- behaviors

These values, beliefs, attitudes, and behaviors are generally unspoken and unwritten, but they help guide how the employees work together.

A company culture is shaped by its **core values**, or a set of guidelines on behaviors that are needed to achieve the vision or purpose of a company. These guidelines are often written in a company's code of conduct as well as provided as the mission statement, which may be posted on the company's public website. A **mission statement** is a formal summary of the aims and values of a company or organization.

There are many informal ways that company culture is expressed. If a company values the environment, for example, then it might stock the employee breakroom with reusable silverware and mugs and provide recycling bins. If a company values collaboration, it may wish to set up open work spaces so that employees can interact more frequently with one another.

During your job search, it is important to find a workplace that aligns well with your own core values and whose company culture you think will be a good fit.

4.6 Module Summary

Your knowledge of pharmacy practice is only part of what it takes to have a successful career as a technician. Your behavior in the field is an integral component and consists of many factors. By learning from your experiences as a student and in an externship, developing healthy self-esteem, and being aware of how others view your professional reputation, your professional image will excel. Displaying leadership qualities, emotional intelligence, adaptability, and accountability will contribute to your advancement to greater positions of responsibility and higher compensation. Practice continual awareness and improvement of these traits, and your chances of success will increase.

 The online course includes additional review and assessment resources.

Professional Communications

LEARNING OBJECTIVES

1   Identify different types of communication. (Section 5.1)

2   Understand the role communication plays in workplace success. (Section 5.1)

3   Understand and practice verbal communication skills. (Section 5.2)

4   Learn the steps of active speaking. (Section 5.2)

5   Understand phone etiquette and interactions. (Section 5.2)

6   Learn the steps of active listening. (Section 5.2)

7   Understand nonverbal communication. (Section 5.3)

8   Learn and practice professional email standards of interaction. (Section 5.4)

9   Identify professional standards of documentation. (Section 5.4)

10 Learn to adjust communication methods to accomodate unique communication needs. (Section 5.5)

11 Identify steps to handle coworker communications. (Section 5.6)

12 Learn how to communicate medication safety concerns. (Section 5.6)

13 Identify steps to handle patient communications. (Section 5.7)

14 Understand the Health Insurance Portability and Accountability Act (HIPAA) and its influence on communication. (Section 5.7)

To view the *ASHP/ACPE Accreditation Standards* addressed in this chapter, refer to Appendix A.

A key part of being successful in the workplace is possessing effective communication skills. According to a recent LinkedIn survey, the top skill set employers seek is communication skills. During your career, you will inevitably encounter difficult situations and hard-to-please coworkers, customers, and patients. You will need to use effective communication skills to arrive at a positive outcome. This means expressing your ideas clearly and logically, making yourself understood, and understanding others.

This module will introduce you to different types of communication and show you how to develop good communication skills. Some of the topics addressed include verbal communication, phone etiquette, active listening and speaking, written communication, effective communication using technology, and communication laws.

5.1 Communication

Communication is a process by which information is exchanged between individuals. There are three types of communication, which will be covered in more depth later in the module:

- **Verbal communication** includes spoken words (what you say and hear).
- **Nonverbal communication** includes body language, facial expressions, hand gestures, etc., (e.g., how you deliver or receive messages).
- **Written communication** includes email, text, professional documentation, and letters (e.g., the words you write).

Communicating effectively can be considered the oil in the engine of the pharmacy, keeping everything running smoothly. Without oil, an engine will seize up and stop working completely.

Using the information and activities provided throughout this module, you will develop communication skills necessary for career success. The first step is to assess your current communication skills.

Self-Reflection:
How Effectively Do You Communicate?

For each statement, answer "always," "sometimes," or "rarely/never." Respond to statements as honestly as possible.

Statement	Always	Sometimes	Rarely/Never
I watch the listener(s) to try to anticipate and deal with problems and confusion when communicating with others.			

Continues…

Statement	Always	Sometimes	Rarely/Never
If I do not understand something, I ask for clarification, even if I think others might view my question as stupid.			
I regularly find that people understand what I tell them.			
When engaging in a conversation, I give the speaker my full attention.			
I consider how others perceive my words and sometimes change the way I say something so that it is better received.			
I consider the feelings of others when speaking, and I sometimes don't speak my mind.			
When people tell me something I don't agree with, I try to first see it from their perspective before responding with how I feel.			
When talking to people, I pay attention to their body language.			
I slow my rate of speech when providing or verifying information.			
I consider cultural and age barriers when talking and listening.			
Before I say something, I think about what the person needs to know and how best to convey that information.			
When trying to resolve a conflict, I pause to think and find something to agree with before stating my difference in perspective.			
Subtotal per column	_____ x5	_____ x3	_____ x1

Tally Your Score: Always = 5 points; Sometimes = 3 points; Rarely/Never = 1 point

Total Score: _____

50 to 60 points: You understand your role as a communicator, both when you send messages and when you receive them. You anticipate problems, and you choose the most effective ways of communicating.

31 to 49 points: You need to keep working on your communication skills. You may not be expressing yourself clearly, and you may not be receiving messages correctly. By paying attention to communication, you can be much more effective at work and enjoy better working relationships.

30 or fewer points: You have poor communication skills and should work quickly and diligently to improve these skills.

Understanding the Benefits of Good Communication Skills

There are many benefits to good communication skills, especially when working in a community pharmacy or institutional setting. Possessing effective communication skills will improve safety for your patients, customer satisfaction, as well as coworker interactions. Being an effective communicator will help make you the type of employee a pharmacy will want to hire.

Improve Safety and Dispensing Efficiency When the pharmacy staff is communicating well, safety is increased, as is the speed of production for medication delivery. For example, if you ask when a patient plans to pick up a medication, you can identify its priority in your fill order. Or if you notice a new opioid prescription without an accompanying laxative, you can communicate it to the pharmacist to see if you should follow up with the prescriber.

Improve Customer Satisfaction A technician in a community setting who does not communicate well with patients can cause them to become angry and frustrated, potentially leading them to take their business elsewhere. A technician who communicates well, on the other hand, can lead to patients telling friends and family how well they were treated, potentially increasing business. Often, good communication forms lasting relationships with patients and allows for easier interactions, even when there are issues, such as insurance challenges.

Improve Coworker Interactions If you get along well with your coworkers, going to work becomes more pleasant. A pharmacy staff works best as a team, and good communication skills contribute positively to building that team.

Developing Good Communication Skills for Employability

Developing effective communication skills will help you find a job and excel in your career. Pharmacies are looking for technicians who are effective communicators. In a job interview, good communication skills can help give you an edge against the competition. Once you have a career in the field, good communication skills can help you keep your job and continue to grow in your career. Communication skills are vital in the pharmacy. You will need to listen to your supervisor's directions, communicate with fellow technicians, and provide excellent customer service.

The time and effort spent to improve your communication skills will help you as you begin your career and will allow you to be a more productive and efficient employee.

5.2 Verbal Communication Skills

Words, and how they are delivered, help patients and coworkers form lasting impressions and opinions of your character. Often, we are unaware of the many factors that affect our speech. In normal interactions with friends and family, we don't need to be as focused on these factors. But knowing these factors and improving them for the professional setting is essential.

Adjusting Pitch, Volume, Tone, and Pace to the Workplace

The pitch, volume, and tone of your voice, as well as pacing, are crucial to successful communication. These factors contribute to your overall professional presence, as well as being important to many aspects of pharmacy technician practice. Whether answering phone calls; talking to nurses, doctors, or patients; or interviewing for your first position, your pitch, volume, and tone can make or break these encounters.

Control Your Pitch **Pitch** is the highness or lowness of the voice based on the frequency of sound waves. A person who speaks in a high-pitched voice may be perceived as immature or overly emotional. A low, gruff, or rough-sounding voice could be mistaken for grumpiness unless the voice is accompanied by a smile and friendly facial expressions and gestures. Those who end their sentences in an upward pitch sound hesitant, or as though they sound like they are asking a question instead of making a statement. Lastly, a person speaking in a monotone voice may be perceived as uninterested or uncaring.

Adjust Your Volume The **volume** of your voice describes how loudly or softly you speak. You will need to strike the right balance between being too loud or too quiet. In a hospital setting, a fellow technician may be working on a difficult IV calculation, or be on the phone with a soft-spoken physician. In either of those cases, talking too loudly can be a distraction to the technician's work. At the same time, speaking too softly to a patient at the window in a community setting will make it hard for them to clearly understand what you are saying. The person will have to strain to hear your words properly and may feel frustrated by the encounter.

Deciding how loudly to speak has to do with the situation and the listener. If you are speaking to someone with some hearing loss, you may have to speak more loudly. If you are speaking of personal medication matters, you may want to draw that person to a quiet corner or office to avoid having to shout out protected health information—which would cause Health Insurance Portability and Accountability Act (HIPAA) compliance issues (discussed later in this module).

Watch Your Tone Equally as important as your pitch and volume is your tone of voice. **Tone** of voice is the attitude conveyed toward your audience through your speech. It is the feeling or mood you communicate. You communicate your attitude in voice patterns, volume, word choices, speed of speech, and emphasis of certain words. Customers and patients generally want a respectful, warm, personal tone, rather than an overly formal approach. A tone of empathy, concern, friendliness, and helpfulness is the most effective in the pharmacy environment.

Practice Tip

Avoid speaking louder to someone who is a non-English speaker. Speaking louder doesn't make it easier for that person to understand you and will draw unwanted attention to your conversation.

Imagine a customer comes in and says that he forgot to take one of his medications and is wondering if it will be a dangerous problem. Consider how he would respond if you said, "You did WHAT?!" or asked calmly, "Can you tell me what happened?"

Though you can't hear these two approaches, you can see on paper the difference in tone when you emphasize the word "what" and ask the question loudly versus asking a basic question in a calm manner. The first example conveys surprise and exasperation. The second option shows more kindness, respect, and concern. "Can you tell me what happened?" is a common phrase to memorize because you can use it often to gather the information needed to provide to the pharmacist for patient counseling.

Pace Your Speech When people talk so fast you cannot catch what they are saying, you must ask them to repeat themselves. Don't repeat this mistake in the pharmacy, especially when the information you are conveying is essential to a patient's health. Adjust your rate of speech to match the listener's abilities. Always watch your listener's reactions. If the listener seems frustrated or puzzled, slow down your pace.

Speaking Actively

Understanding the mechanics of verbal communication helps build the skills of becoming an active speaker. **Active speaking** is conveying your message with awareness as to how the receiver is interpreting your information, being able to adapt as necessary. The following sections address seven key principles of effectively delivering a message (as the sender/speaker):

1. Be positive.
2. Be humble.
3. Be patient.
4. Be tactful.
5. Be honest.
6. Avoid generalizations.
7. Check understanding.

> "Active speaking is conveying your message with awareness as to how the receiver is interpreting your information..."

These speaking skills are used in everyday life at different times. However, few of us use them consistently. Being aware of these skills enables you to use them more proficiently.

Be Positive Try to be cheerful and smile whenever dealing with others. Add a compliment or statement of gratitude when appropriate. Acknowledge similar points of view whenever possible.

Be Humble Be mindful of the message you are communicating. Avoid arrogant, boasting statements or ones that put others down. You can still make definitive statements of content and perspective, but make them in the context of providing information to use for dialog and consideration, not to shut down other's perspectives.

Be Patient It can be challenging to wait for people to finish their sentences, especially if those sentences spark a thought. This skill requires patience. Interrupting speakers almost always leads to upset and frustration.

Be Tactful **Tact** is having sensitivity to what is proper and appropriate in dealing with others, including the ability to speak or act without offending them. For instance, some questions are not tactful, appropriate, or strategic to ask, such as asking what a person's salary is. If you ask yourself, "I wonder whether I should say/write that?" then the answer is almost always no.

Be Honest Answer questions with honesty. This does not mean that you should be brutally honest with people—just sincere. Brutal honesty is often hurtful and usually unnecessary to convey the message. Tact is very useful here. For example, if the person responsible for purchasing the medications for a hospital pharmacy asks your opinion of a new ordering process, it is best to give an honest reply, even if it is not necessarily what the person wants to hear. But also consider that it is more important to protect your working relationship than to deeply criticize a process you may not agree with. You might say, "I like the new protocol for back-ordered medication. The turnaround time isn't as fast as I would like, but I understand that it is an element that is hard to control." Don't elaborate on or embellish criticism. If people are really interested in your feedback, they will question you further about the features you do not appreciate.

Avoid Generalizations Many times, when we are in a hurry, we use very general language to describe something. "Could you please help the heart patient while I handle this phone call?" This type of request would lead to follow-up questions by the receiver, which would take more time to explain rather than being helpful. Consider instead saying, "Could you please assist Mrs. Fredericks with her medication, which is written here, while I handle the call on line one?"

Check Understanding Make sure to check in with the person to whom you are speaking with to make sure the message was properly understood. People may be listening, but you can't always tell if they understand your main point. You can fix that by asking confirming questions, such as, "Did that make sense?" "Do you think that could work?" or "Would you be able to do that?" If there are several directions, such as providing the steps for the proper dosing for a child or a list of medications to retrieve from the storeroom, you may ask someone, "Can you please repeat those steps back, so we make sure not to miss any?"

Honing Your Telephone Etiquette and Skills

One of the most practical applications of technicians' verbal communication skills is their telephone interactions. A large portion of a technician's workflow involves answering phone calls. Being efficient and effective in this area is a very good way to demonstrate your competence as a technician.

When making a phone call, you may have encountered unprofessional phone etiquette, such as:

- The person answering the phone is difficult to understand.
- The voicemail message consists of only a few words, such as "leave a message."
- Loud background noises prevent you from hearing the other person.
- The person you've called sounds annoyed when answering.

These examples leave you with a negative impression of the person or business that you've called.

Professional phone skills can be organized into four components:

1. answering properly
2. listening intently
3. remaining calm
4. returning a call and leaving a message

As more business is conducted online, many people are losing basic telephone etiquette skills. To build professional phone skills, first consider your current phone skills.

 Self-Reflection:
Consider Your Phone Skills

For each of the statements, answer "always," "sometimes," or "rarely/never." Respond to statements as honestly as possible.

When I talk on the phone, I think that I …	Always	Sometimes	Rarely/Never
sound friendly.			
convey interest.			
am clear—there's no mumbling or confusing directions.			
sound professional.			
ask for permission when I need to put someone on hold.			
give undivided attention.			

Continues…

When I talk on the phone, I think that I …	Always	Sometimes	Rarely/Never
do not interrupt.			
do not have side conversations.			
am polite and say "please" and "thank you."			
express understanding and empathy.			
resolve issues.			
minimize background noise.			
listen to a caller's frustration and anger without matching it.			
sound knowledgeable about pharmacy.			
say "thank you" and then wait for the listener to hang up.			
Subtotal per column	_____ x5	_____ x3	_____ x1

Tally Your Score: Always = 5 points; Sometimes = 3 points; Rarely/Never = 1 point

Total Score: _____

61 to 75 points: You have excellent telephone skills and manners.

51 to 60 points: Your current level of telephone skills and manners is satisfactory; however, there is room for improvement.

31 to 50 points: Your current level of telephone skills and manners is below average, and you need to work on these skills.

30 or fewer points: You have poor telephone skills and manners and should work quickly and diligently to improve your skills.

Consider your performance. In which phone skills are you most confident? Which will require more practice?

Answer the Phone Properly The importance of answering the phone for a pharmacy should never be underestimated. We become the face of our business every time we answer the phone. How that experience is handled is a direct reflection of the business's attitude toward customer service and a reflection of your professionalism. Whether that telephone conversation is with a customer or one of your peers, ensuring that every phone interaction is positive is important.

Using the phone takes away your ability to communicate using nonverbal cues (such as facial expressions), so you must adopt certain techniques that convey your interest in their calls and desire to assist them. Answering the phone right away with an appropriate greeting conveys interest.

Effective Answering Techniques When the phone rings, stop what you are doing and prepare yourself for the call. Take a moment to slow down your rate of speech and speak clearly. Your tone of voice must demonstrate to callers that you are upbeat and eager to take their information or help with questions. If callers hear more than a few rings, they may assume that you are either not available or are busy. Common etiquette is to answer a phone by the third ring, even if it is to ask the caller to be placed on hold.

Appropriate Greetings Always answer the phone by stating the name of the pharmacy and your name. For example, you might say, "Thank you for calling Johnson Pharmacy. This is Mary. How can I help you?" Or, if answering your personal phone, you might say, "Good morning, this is Isla Perez speaking; how can I help you?"

"Smiling projects friendliness and warmth and makes speaking at a normal rate of speed easier."

A great deal of research has been done about people being able to sense a smile through tone of voice on the phone. Equally, people can sense a frown. Smiling projects friendliness and warmth and makes speaking at a normal rate of speed easier.

Try to determine the caller's name early and attempt to use it again during the call. Doing so indicates that you are paying attention to the details of the call.

Leave Effective Phone Messages Knowing how to leave a professional voicemail will reflect positively on you and your pharmacy. Planning ahead, speaking slowly, and ending the message professionally will help you to leave effective phone messages.

Message Content Before you pick up the phone to call someone, pause for a moment and summarize in your mind the purpose of the call in one or two sentences. Be prepared to leave a concise message. Begin every call by introducing yourself. You might say, "Hello. This is Ken Wantanabe returning your call regarding setting up an interview for the pharmacy technician position." Speak slowly when leaving a message. It can be very frustrating when retrieving messages if one must replay it repeatedly to hear the necessary information.

Professional Goodbye End by giving your contact information, and always say "thank you." It is a good idea to repeat your telephone number and slowly spell any words that may be uncommonly spelled.

Listening Actively

Communication is a two-way street. It is not just about how well you convey your message, but also how well you receive the message of whomever you are communicating with. This requires you to listen well in addition to speaking well.

According to Businessdictionary.com, **active listening** is "the act of mindfully hearing and attempting to comprehend the meaning of words spoken by another in a conversation or speech."

Active listening helps to minimize misunderstandings and miscommunication. Although misunderstandings are a part of life, your ability to recognize and correct these misunderstandings elevates you from a good communicator to a superior communicator.

People often listen passively, letting their minds wander even as they are watching the speaker. They are only partially present and not fully engaged in what the person is saying.

To be an active listener, you must apply some skills that let the speaker know that you are engaged, receptive, and interested in the conversation. These skills are particularly important in serving a patient, taking a phone call, conducting a job interview, or having a difficult conversation.

The practices for active listening include the following:

- putting away or turning off electronics
- paying and showing attention
- having attentive, open posture and body language
- asking for clarification as needed
- reiterating what the speaker says
- showing empathy
- providing a thoughtful response

Put Away Electronics The most inconsiderate action most people commit in today's world is using electronics during conversations. Glancing at your phone, reading emails, checking text messages, and working on a computer while conversing are signs to others that you don't have time for them and find little value in what they are saying.

If you must use an electronic device during a phone call, let the speaker know in advance that you'll be taking notes or checking medication information on the computer. This way, the person will not misinterpret sounds.

Pay Attention Give speakers your undivided attention by looking them directly in the eye. Focus on what the person is saying without thinking how you might respond. Let the person know you are paying attention by interjecting comments, such as "I understand," "That's interesting," and "I see." You can also use simple noises, such as "uh-huh" or "hmm."

If appropriate, taking notes is a nonverbal way of acknowledging the speaker. Notes are also important if you are being given directions with more than a few steps, especially if they involve medication accuracy and patient safety. Do not rely on your memory.

Have Open Posture and Body Language Maintain a relaxed and open posture when listening to someone speak. Don't cross your arms. If possible, squarely face the speaker. Avoid slouching because this pose may indicate to the speaker that you're bored. Having an open and relaxed posture will not only help the speaker remain calm but will also show that you are open to the speaker's message.

Ask for Clarification as Needed Open-ended questions cannot be answered with a simple "yes" or "no" response. Questions beginning with "what," "why," or "how" are open-ended questions. They require speakers to provide more detail and elaborate on their message. Asking open-ended questions demonstrates to speakers that you are genuine in your desire to fully understand the message they are trying to convey.

Reiterate What the Speaker Says Paraphrasing or restating what the speaker has said in your own words lets them know that you are listening. It also gives that person the opportunity to clarify the message. To be clear, reiterating is not repeating word for word what the speaker said. Provide a summary of what you think are the key points to be sure you heard what the person meant.

Show Empathy **Empathy** is understanding and sharing another person's experiences and emotions or having the ability to imagine someone else's feelings. This ability to make others feel understood allows powerful communicators to redirect others toward finding solutions rather than blaming. You can express this by simply listening. You may also say you understand why they think or feel that way.

"This ability to make others feel understood allows powerful communicators to redirect others toward finding solutions rather than blaming"

Provide a Thoughtful Response Only after you're certain you understand the real problem and what is needed should you offer a response. In many situations, people are looking for some specific action, change, or solution to a problem, particularly at work. Patients want solutions to their medication therapy questions. In this case, you can refer them to the pharmacist. They may want insurance issues resolved, which you can help them with. To effectively transition, one method is to state, "That is a question that the pharmacist can answer best; let me get her for you."

Build Rapport Responding with a story of a time something similar happened helps to build rapport. **Rapport** is when individuals or groups understand one another and communicate well.

Find Common Ground If you and the speaker have differences in approach, opinion, or belief, your response can be to sum up the areas of agreement and those in which you have a different perspective. You can outline why you see things differently and decide next actions based on what the situation requires.

> ### Think It Through: Considering Other's Listening Skills
> Think of one person who has had an influence in your life. Identify which active listening skills they demonstrated or possessed.

5.3 Nonverbal Communication Skills

Many elements comprise nonverbal communication. In every direct interaction, what you are saying verbally is one part being conveyed, while nonverbal actions convey their own message. Nonverbal communication can have a great influence on the outcome of any discussion.

Even though we are not always consciously aware of nonverbal acts, they influence any communication you engage in. It is often said that while people may not verbally always tell the truth, body language rarely lies because it is not consciously used. This is why poker players have "tells," or physical indicators of what kind of hand they may have been dealt. As a technician, if you develop and pay attention to the nonverbal signals of yourself and others, it can be a very useful tool.

Paying Attention to Facial Expressions and Gestures

People's faces many times convey the emotions they are feeling, even if their words do not. Pay attention to unconscious reactions, such as eye rolling, expressions of noninterest (or interest), and eye contact. This will allow you to adjust your communication accordingly. Also develop an awareness of your own reactions during conversation.

Using your hands and arms to gesture while talking is common. Some use it to a greater or lesser degree. It can convey excitement or passion for a subject. Professional communicators observe the level of gestures used by the person they are speaking to and adjust their own motions to match. This forms a level of unconscious similarity and can enhance the dialogue.

Another example of a gesture is folded arms. This is commonly associated with closing yourself off or creating a barrier between yourself and another speaker. Nonverbal communication is contextual, so be aware that folding arms could also mean the person is physically cold and trying to stay warm.

Considering Distance and Positioning

Everyone has a **personal bubble**, a physical space that is defined as being too close. Being inside someone's bubble can cause discomfort and severely affect communications. Everyone's personal bubble is different. A great communicator is aware of this and closely observes where that boundary is. If you accidentally get into someone's personal space, the person will move to create a safe distance if possible. Be aware of this and mark the boundary. If you are already in a very small area (which is common in pharmacies), do your best to use the distance that is available to reduce tension.

The position of one's body is also a large element of nonverbal signals. A slouched posture can indicate disinterest, tiredness, or laziness. A straight posture conversely can convey alertness, interest, and high energy. If you are speaking with people who do not turn their feet or body to face you, it can be an indication that they do not want to engage in conversation. Take note of that and do not take up more time than is necessary to deliver your message.

EXPAND YOUR KNOWLEDGE

History of Nonverbal Communication

Nonverbal communication has been studied since Charles Darwin's publication *The Expression of the Emotions in Man and Animals*. We convey so much through our facial expressions and gestures. Some other lesser-known forms of nonverbal communication include eye gaze (how often you maintain eye contact, the dilation of your pupils, and how frequently you blink), haptics (using touch to convey care, concern, or even power), and appearance. Consider how different forms of nonverbal communication influence your communication in this article by Kendra Cherry, "Type of Nonverbal Communication." https://SSPharm.ParadigmEducation.com/NonverbalCommunication

5.4 Written Communication Skills

Besides in-person communication skills, you need to practice professional written communications. These can include emails and other professional documentation, such as faxes and refill authorizations. The power of the written word cannot be underestimated. It is more permanent than verbal communications, and care must be taken when using this medium in a professional setting.

Using Email Professionally

Your email behavior at work has the potential to sabotage your reputation both personally and professionally. Poorly written emails can offend or confuse customers or colleagues. Employees can be terminated for using email inappropriately. Consider everything you write in email to be potentially public, easily forwarded to others at work, or posted on social media without your knowledge or consent.

Avoid Common Email Pitfalls There are many ways to fail at writing professional emails. By being aware of the potential pitfalls, your emails can reflect the level of professionalism that is desired by employers. Use the following strategies to prevent common mistakes when composing emails.

Proofreading Always edit your emails to ensure that you sound professional. Use grammar and spell check and then read everything again because autocorrect can introduce errors, and words with multiple meanings can be missed. Grammar and spell check do not catch everything.

Message Content Begin with the correct professional title and greeting to the receiver. Add a pleasantry—a warm greeting, thank you for an earlier action or email, or a compliment. This simple statement will go a long way in opening the door for the recipient's willingness to listen to the message you are about to deliver. Keep messages brief and to the point. Emails should cover only one topic or request whenever possible.

Abbreviations and Emoticons Avoid using text abbreviations of any kind in a professional email. Most business email shouldn't include emoticons. This can be a difficult habit to break, as it is so common in text messaging communications today, but emoticons are often perceived as unprofessional.

Professional Signature Include a signature that has your contact information to ensure that people know who you are as well as the best ways to communicate with you. This signature should include your name, title, website (if applicable), and relevant phone numbers.

Manage Email Effectively There are some rules of engagement when it comes to responding to emails in a professional manner. Responding in a timely manner, avoiding forwarding and group email, using carbon copy effectively, and practicing caution around chain letters and other junk mail all contribute to professional email management.

Replies You want to acknowledge that you received a message even if you don't have the full answer or haven't completed the requested action. Let the sender know that you saw the message and provide an estimate for when you expect to reply with the information requested.

Email Forwards It is considered rude to forward an email to another party without seeking and obtaining permission from the original sender. If you cannot get permission, then you should summarize the information in your own words.

Group Email Send group email only when it's useful to every recipient. Use the "Reply all" button only if you have something important to add. Group email recipients can get quite annoyed to open an email that says only "Thank you!" or "Great!" If you need to send a response, reply only to the original sender.

Bcc and Cc Options Bcc (blind carbon copy) and cc (carbon copy) are options you can select when sending emails to more than one recipient. Cc sends a copy of the correspondence to a third party (and both the sender and recipient see the extra recipients). Use cc only when a third party is directly involved or has requested inclusion. Bcc sends a copy of the correspondence to the third party without the knowledge of the main recipient. The bcc option can appear secretive and should be avoided in most cases. However, if you must mail to a large distribution list, then it is appropriate to use. It protects the privacy of the recipients and prevents all the recipients from having to see a large list of email addresses.

Chain Letters or Spam Work email should be limited to work-related subjects. If you receive non-work-related emails from a colleague, ask that person to send such emails to your personal email account.

Documenting Professionally

Proper documentation is crucial in pharmacy practice. **Documentation** is material that provides official information or evidence or that serves as a record. It is necessary to be able to provide a paper trail of actions regarding the care of a patient. Some of the most important reasons for documentation are improving patient care and outcomes, protecting against legal liability, following laws and regulations, and aiding in data analysis. Examples can be taking note of a refill authorization over the phone, completing a compounding log, or even recording a technician's initials on a label to identify who filled it. Your training once hired will introduce you to the specific policies and procedures required in a given setting. There are some key general principles to remember, however, when documenting things in the pharmacy, such as logging pertinent information and correcting errors properly.

Communicate Pertinent Information One saying in health care is, "If you didn't document it, it didn't happen." Identify the pertinent information that must be recorded for a given procedure. For example, for a telephone refill authorization, a technician must record the full name and position title of the person authorizing the refill. If it is for a controlled substance, some states require the ICD-10 diagnosis code of the condition be listed, and a technician may have to ask for that during the communication. Another example is the information needed when batching a compounded preparation. There is typically a log sheet that requires several pieces of data to be documented accurately, such as lot number and expiration date. Always find out what needs to be documented for a given interaction or procedure and do so in a legible manner. It is not proper documentation if it cannot be read later.

Handle Errors in Documentation Properly There is always a chance that you might make an error during documentation. This could be the wrong number written on a narcotic log sheet or a misspelling of a name on a refill authorization form. The proper method to correct an error is to mark a single line through it with the correction written after it. The purpose is to see what the error was and understand it—not hide it. You should never scribble something out or use correction fluid when making a correction.

5.5 Special Patient Population Communications

As a pharmacy technician, you will encounter a wide variety of customers, patients, and coworkers. Many will have challenges that affect how you communicate with them, in both verbal and written forms. Cultural issues surrounding communication will be discussed in Module 6. However, communication considerations for patients with physical or mental impairments, or patients experiencing economic hardship are covered in the sections below.

Accommodating for Physical and Mental Impairments

When patients have physical or mental impairments, they require special accommodations by pharmacy personnel. These communications require empathy and compassion, as well as patience, to be handled correctly. You will encounter many different types of impairments; being aware of them beforehand is the first step to being able to handle them effectively.

Communicate Effectively with Patients with Visual and Hearing Impairments A pair of customer reading glasses or large-print or Braille materials are helpful to have on hand at the pharmacy register. You may assist customers by filling a plastic drug organizer with the week's or months' worth of medication for them. Customers who are hard of hearing may benefit from a slow, deliberate, short discourse (for lip reading) or—if they are deaf—from sign language or written instructions.

Communicate Effectively with Patients with Mental and Physical Challenges If you are interacting with a patient who struggles with comprehension or cannot move easily to where you are, be particularly understanding and accommodating. Provide directions about medication use or payment in simple, clear, direct terms without slang or jargon. Check often for understanding. For patients with physical impairments, pharmacy personnel should make every effort to accommodate their needs. These accommodations may include recommending drive-through service, using nonchildproof container lids, helping obtain items from shelves, or ensuring their comfort while waiting for their medications to be prepared.

Accommodating for Economic Hardship

Hard economic times and rising healthcare costs have made it increasingly difficult for patients to afford medications and other forms of medical treatment. Pharmacy staff members should be empathic to these patients' needs and offer alternatives for payment assistance. Often prescription discount cards and plans may be available.

> **Think It Through: How Do You React to Communication Barriers?**
> Brainstorm an instance of when a communication barrier caused a problem in your own life. Write a summary of what happened. Then identify steps you could take to avoid making (or encountering) this communication error in the future.

5.6 Coworker Communication Considerations

Despite all the effort of practicing active listening, speaking clearly, using open nonverbal communication, and writing professional correspondence, conflicts can still arise. Knowing how to approach these scenarios, both as a speaker and listener, requires certain skills. These skills can decrease tension and increase the possibility of positive outcomes. These are not only helpful in workplace situations but also in personal interactions.

Preventing Conversations from Escalating

Many communication interactions have the potential to escalate because of the content being discussed, the attitudes of the parties involved, and the stress of the situation. Several general tips and tricks can help prevent or deescalate a conversation between coworkers.

Save Face People can get defensive when they feel they are being personally blamed or attacked in a conversation. To help avoid defensiveness, use "I" or "we" in statements rather than "you." Using "you" statements places blame on others and implies that they are at fault or don't understand. For example, say you work with a person who likes to get straight to the point and you prefer detailed explanations. Instead of saying, "You talk really fast; could you slow down?" you could say, "I'm concerned that I may make a mistake if I don't get all the details correct. Could you please explain it a little slower, so I can better understand what you need me to do?" This type of interaction shifts the accountability to you rather than the other person.

Avoid Trigger Words Nothing will escalate a miscommunication faster than the use of words like "always" and "never." These and others are commonly referred to as *trigger words*. For example, when you say, "You never restock the pill vials," the receiver immediately becomes defensive, which isn't the point of the statement. Maybe the person just hasn't restocked lately. A more effective way to express the same message would be to say, "I know you were busy last week, but the pill vials are running empty. Maybe we can find a way to shift some responsibilities to help with that." The person may still disagree but is more likely to focus on finding a solution.

Redirect Focus When you are working with others on a team, problems may arise; when they do, it is important to address the actual problems, not someone's ideas or the person themselves. This follows the same concept of saving face. For example, someone suggests an idea that you feel has many negative consequences that aren't being considered. You may say, "I can see what you are suggesting, but let me just play the devil's advocate for the moment. If we do this, then 'xyz' may happen." You are not trying to criticize the other person's idea but are providing additional information that needs to be considered from another point of view. When an interaction falls into a personal attack against you, bring the conversation back to addressing the problem. For instance, you could say, "I think we should focus on finding a solution, not assigning blame," or, "There are many reasons why this problem arose, so let's try to address them." Ask yourself, "What is the real issue? How can I address it specifically?"

Summarize Common Ground You can settle things down by summing up the common ground in what has been shared. People listen better when they see that someone has understood and agreed with aspects of what they have tried to convey. If you can say, "I agree with you in this," or, "That makes sense," then you can follow with the areas in which you have different perspectives.

Be Humble Nothing can oppress real listening or understanding more than acting as if you know everything. This often stems from an insecurity in position or status. There are always other perspectives that have relevance. Even if you do know a large amount about a subject, you do not have to prove it by stating it.

Seek Win-Win Solutions Make it clear to the listener that you want the best solution for everyone. Look for ways that everyone comes away with some benefit. "OK, let's see how we can find something that works for all of us."

Take Criticism Constructively If you receive constructive criticism, take it well. A professional considers criticism as counsel that can help you do better. In your job reviews, you will be given a list of expectations and suggestions. If you take these in the right spirit of humility and wanting to improve, these reviews can often help you grow and succeed in your career goals.

Addressing Medication Safety Concerns and Errors

One of the core tenets of pharmacy practice is medication safety. While many systems and protocols are in place to prevent them, errors still occur. Sometimes those same systems may have flaws that need to be corrected. Many errors that occur are human.

Accountability is defined as an obligation or willingness to accept responsibility or to account for one's actions. As a pharmacy technician, this holds true not only to yourself but also to your coworkers, supervisors, and the pharmacy. By holding everyone and everything accountable, medication safety is increased. When errors occur, it is best to communicate and demonstrate accountability.

Consider Institutional Accountability Sometimes a policy or procedure in a pharmacy is not working or is not working as well as it could. There may be elements that allow for errors to occur. Often it is a pharmacy technician who raises the flag on these issues. Pharmacy technicians should be encouraged to question whether a process or procedure could be modified or improved or to offer suggestions on how to do so.

The best practice for how to communicate these observations is to do so in a respectful manner. First state the problem you have observed and why you think it might lead to an error. Most likely, you will want to alert a more senior technician or a pharmacist. Allow that person to explain the process. Perhaps there is a valid reason it is done the way it is. If not, then either offer a suggestion on how to modify the process or ask if there is a way to do so.

Take Personal Accountability If you discover a mistake you made, immediately take steps to correct it, and notify the appropriate coworker, whether it is the lead technician or the pharmacist. This allows others to learn from your mistake and not make it again. Often, we are afraid, especially when starting a new position, to admit mistakes. We worry mistakes make us look bad to our employers. However, the opposite is true. If a mistake or error is discovered by someone else and brought to your attention, accept it graciously. An appropriate response could be, "I am very sorry for making this mistake, and

Work Wise

Everyone makes mistakes—pharmacists, technicians, and patients alike. What will set you apart is how you accept responsibility for and correct the mistakes you make.

Career Readiness & Externships: Soft Skills for Pharmacy Technicians

Words to Live By

In any workplace, there are mistakes, and then there are MISTAKES. These larger mistakes in pharmacy are typically very expensive or potentially very harmful to a patient. These can include damaging or ruining an expensive medication or making a severe medication fill error. I had one of these MISTAKES in the retail setting—I filled a medication order incorrectly, which was very costly. My managing pharmacist was understandably upset.

I said in a humble tone, "I am very sorry for the error. I realize that I will make mistakes, but I promise you that I will make each mistake only once." It was an admission of my fallibility but also a commitment to performing better moving forward. Work hard to ensure that every mistake is one you learn from.

–Mark Brunton, MSHE, CPhT

I will work to prevent it from happening again. Thank you for letting me know." Depending on the nature of the mistake, it might be useful to take a written note for future reference.

Handle Coworker Accountability It is almost certain that during your career as a technician, you will catch an error made by a coworker or notice them doing something incorrectly. This can be a delicate situation. It can be hard to be told by a coworker that you made a mistake, especially if that coworker is newer or younger. There are ways to handle an error observation with tact and achieve a positive outcome.

Remember the previously mentioned tactics for coworker communications, such as saving face and avoiding trigger words. Do not tell your coworkers, "You made a mistake"; rather, question the procedure or nature of the error, allowing them to discover the mistake and correct it. You might say, "Is that ER or SR for that medication?" or, "How far do we have to be inside the hood to make IVs?" By asking as if for your own knowledge, it saves face yet communicates the error to the coworker.

If there is ever a situation in which a coworker is blatantly disregarding your communication, unwilling to take accountability, and putting patient safety at risk, notifying a supervisor is the next course of action.

Examine Supervisor Accountability Every pharmacist is considered a technician supervisor. Pharmacists have an advanced degree, are the ones who counsel patients, and are ultimately responsible for every medication that leaves the pharmacy. But pharmacists also make mistakes, and it may be a technician who discovers them. The best pharmacists are those who recognize and rely on technicians as a second set of eyes to catch errors and bring concerns to their attention. But some may get defensive or dismissive of being questioned by their technicians.

The same protocols for coworker accountability apply in these interactions. But what if a pharmacist does not acknowledge the error? It is entirely possible to just let the pharmacist continue, feeling as if you've done your due diligence. But what if there is a potential for a serious medication error to occur? It can be a difficult situation, but using the skills you have learned will help you to communicate that everyone makes mistakes, and patient safety is everyone's goal.

WORKPLACE WISDOM

Communicating Errors with the Pharmacist

A technician at a long-term care pharmacy noticed a potential error in a medication fill. When she brought it to the pharmacist's attention, the pharmacist said, "No, it's fine; I checked it." The technician was very sure there was an error and went back a little while later. The technician said, "I really think there is a mistake with Vance Donaldson's medication that we need to fix." The pharmacist reiterated that it was fine and became irritated with the technician for asking again. The technician asked the other pharmacist on duty, "Could you just double-check me on this prescription? I want to make sure it's safe." The other pharmacist saw the error and corrected it. Later that day, the original pharmacist apologized to the technician.

5.7 Patient Communication Considerations

You will often be the bearer of bad news to patients, informing them of such things as an insurance claim denial, an expensive copayment, or an out–of–stock medication. You must also consider patient privacy in every communication you have with patients. Communicating effectively and safely with patients is one of the toughest challenges you will face as a pharmacy technician but mastering these skills will help you throughout your career.

Communicating Problems and Solutions

One of the first steps in resolving patient challenges is to explain why something will not work. Then communicate other options. For example, take the extra time to explain why a prescription cannot be filled or why it can be only partially filled or why it costs so much. Patients can tolerate inconvenient or disheartening news when the reasons are explained, then you can lay out solutions. If a patient needs an out-of-stock medication, check with your supervising pharmacist and then offer to call neighboring pharmacies to find the medication. If another pharmacy has the medication in stock, arrange for the customer to pick up the prescription at that location. If there is an insurance problem, offer to call the patient's insurance company to find a resolution or call the company later and advise the patient of the outcome. A discount coupon can be offered for many expensive medications.

Handling Angry Customers

Be prepared—you will encounter angry customers in your career. Angry customers are a part of customer service. In pharmacy, however, they may be angry for reasons unrelated to you or the pharmacy visit. A patient may have just received a bad prognosis on an existing disease. Perhaps the patient has spent the last 16 hours in the emergency room. Perhaps a couple has recently lost their jobs and health insurance. Or maybe the person is just having a bad day—we have all been there.

It can be difficult to respond to an angry patient without becoming defensive or escalating the situation, especially without a method to help defuse while remaining calm. LEAD, described below, is a strategy to help you do just that.

Using LEAD Use the acronym LEAD as a reminder of how to respond to complaints: listen, explain why it happened, acknowledge the issues involved, and then discuss to decide what to do (see Figure 5.1).

Figure 5.1 LEAD Is the Way to Handle Angry People

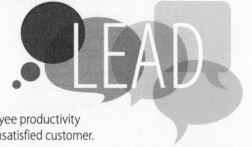

L–**Listen** to the customer

E–**Explain** why it happened

A–**Acknowledge** that it is a legitimate problem

D–**Discuss** to decide how to resolve the issue, and thank the customer

Studies have demonstrated a 20% increase in employee productivity when using similar protocol to handle an angry or unsatisfied customer.

Understanding Patient Confidentiality and Communications

The **Health Insurance Portability and Accountability Act (HIPAA)** regulates access to insurance as well as the privacy of patient information. HIPAA is the reason such strict policies and procedures for confidentiality exist in the pharmacy profession. Violating these regulations can result in hefty fines and, depending on the severity, incarceration.

The national pharmacy chain CVS paid a $2.25 million settlement to the Department of Health and Human Services and submitted a detailed corrective action process due to a HIPAA violation. It was discovered that labels from prescription vials, as well as old prescriptions, were being disposed of in unsecured dumpsters that were accessible to the public.

The confidentiality of patient information can be compromised both verbally and in writing. Assume that all conversations are to be kept confidential regarding patient protected health information (PHI). Even topics that seem insignificant to you may be considered highly personal or private to another person.

You must protect PHI constantly and protect the pharmacy's reputation and customer service standards in every interaction. Digital transmission and fax security are two areas of communication that must be controlled to be HIPAA compliant.

Consider Digital Transmission Issues You will be required to electronically transmit patient PHI to many different parties, including healthcare practitioners, pharmacy personnel, and third-party insurance companies. All such transmissions are protected by state and federal laws. They must be transmitted through software encryption and security systems that fit HIPAA guidelines.

Examine Fax Security Issues Sending medical or prescription information via fax is a common pharmacy practice, especially for refill authorizations from a physician's office. You must carefully monitor faxes to ensure that the original faxing documents and transmissions are not accessible to people outside of the chain of care of the patient, such as other patients or nonpharmacy employees. Faxed information is intended only for personnel of the pharmacy or medical office to which it was sent. If an inadvertent fax was transmitted to the wrong number, the sender must be notified, and the protected information returned or destroyed immediately.

5.8 Module Summary

Professional communications with patients, coworkers, and supervisors is at the heart of what makes a pharmacy run smoothly. When you can do it effectively, you are a valuable resource to the team.

Communications can be difficult and require alertness and awareness. Communicating effectively also requires empathy for others when they struggle to be understood and for yourself when you miscommunicate or don't feel understood. Mastering communication enables you to resolve conflict. Thus, you can build trust and respect not only for yourself but also for your employer.

 The online course includes additional review and assessment resources.

Multicultural Awareness & Cultural Competency

LEARNING OBJECTIVES

1 Become familiar with stereotypes and how to manage their influence on interactions. (Section 6.1)

2 Describe the importance of multicultural awareness and cultural competency in the pharmacy setting. (Section 6.1)

3 Become familiar with the cultural considerations for different ethnic groups and coworkers. (Section 6.2)

4 Identify Eastern vs. Western medicine and the influence they have on each other. (Section 6.2)

5 Describe the cultural considerations for different religions. (Section 6.3)

6 Identify the roles of the pharmacy professional with transgender and other sexual orientation and gender identity demographics. (Section 6.4)

7 Identify best practices for communicating in a culturally competent way. (Section 6.5)

To view the *ASHP/ACPE Accreditation Standards* addressed in this chapter, refer to Appendix A.

n today's pharmacy workplace, you will encounter people from a wide range of backgrounds. In the community setting, the patients you interact with will be of many different demographics. In the institutional setting, your coworkers, physicians, and other healthcare professionals will also have many different ethnic, religious, and cultural backgrounds.

The United States is becoming more ethnically and racially diverse, which poses increased challenges to interacting competently with individuals whose backgrounds may differ.

According to 2016 US Census Bureau estimates, the US population was composed of the racial categories seen in Figure 6.1.

Figure 6.1 Racial Categories in the United States

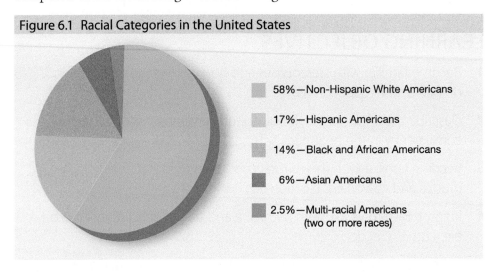

- 58%—Non-Hispanic White Americans
- 17%—Hispanic Americans
- 14%—Black and African Americans
- 6%—Asian Americans
- 2.5%—Multi-racial Americans (two or more races)

You must be sensitive to and respectful of differences in culture, religion, language, age, abilities, sexual orientation, and other backgrounds. To provide the best care to all your patients, as well as to cooperate with colleagues in the workplace, you will need to acquire the skills of cultural competence.

6.1 Multicultural Awareness and Cultural Competency

To understand what is meant by multicultural awareness and cultural competency, it is important to have a clear definition of culture itself. The term **culture** is defined by the United Nations Educational, Scientific, and Cultural Organization (UNESCO) as "a set of distinctive spiritual, material, intellectual and emotional features of society or a social group and that it encompasses, in addition to art and literature, lifestyles, ways of living together, value systems, traditions and beliefs." Although many consider race or ethnicity when they think about culture, it can also include age, religion, disability status, socioeconomics, gender, and sexual orientation.

Figure 6.2 Iceberg Metaphor of Cultural Identity

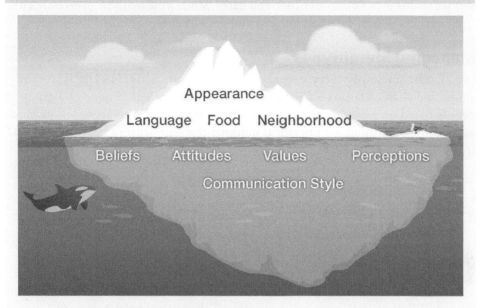

Source: *What Language Does Your Patient Hurt In?* 3e

Social scientist Edward T. Hall compared culture to an iceberg (as seen in Figure 6.2). On the top of a person's cultural iceberg are physical features, manner of dress, native language, accent in speaking English, traditional foods, and neighborhood composition and location. Underneath the visible level are the beliefs, attitudes, values, and perceptions of the person.

Diversity means a broad range of things and can refer to differences in types of people, foods, toys, tools, books, etc.

Multicultural means many cultural groups, whereas **multicultural awareness** refers to the understanding of, appreciation of, and sensitivity to the experiences, values, and lifestyles of people from different backgrounds. A keener understanding of the dimensions that make up another individual or group's diversity will allow you to develop a sense of value and appreciation for a wider subset of cultural values, whether or not you personally identify with them. This multicultural awareness allows you to interact more skillfully in both personal and professional areas of your life, as you interact with friends, family members, acquaintances, patients, and customers.

Cultural competence is defined as the ability of healthcare providers to recognize the social, cultural, and linguistic needs of patients, then deliver the appropriate services that meet those needs. Possessing cultural competence skills will serve you as you begin your career as a pharmacy technician.

Knowing more about a patient's culture will help you provide higher-quality service and shows a customer that you care. When you work to overcome cultural barriers you make every patient and coworker feel at ease.

Managing Stereotypes

We all subconsciously carry stereotypes in our head. A **stereotype** is an over-simplified characteristic of a group of people. It is a generic image of a group of people based on patterns, word-of-mouth stories, prejudiced attitudes, culture assumptions, opinions, or uncritical judgments about isolated incidents blown into sweeping generalizations.

Self-Reflection:
What Stereotypes Do You Have?

The first step in developing cultural competence is to develop self-awareness of your own beliefs, values, stereotypes, and biases. Consider your answers to the following questions.

- Are you religious?
  - If you are religious, what are your feelings about the beliefs and practices of other religions?
  - If you are not religious, what are your feelings about those who are?
- What are your thoughts about alternative forms of health care, such as homeopathic practitioners, herbalists, and shamans?
- How do you express your gender identity?
- How would you respond to a patient whose gender identity was not immediately apparent?
- How would you respond to a patient who refused to look you in the eye?
- How would you react to a colleague who frequently spoke a language other than English in the workplace?

Everyone has biases, but everyone is entitled to respect. A conscious awareness of your own personal stereotypes and biases allows you to challenge the basis and validity of those assumptions, which may lead to greater self-awareness and capacity to accept, recognize, and even embrace the value of the differences that exist in those around you. Equally important is that awareness will help drive your behaviors as you try to keep them from negatively influencing how you treat those with whom you serve and work.

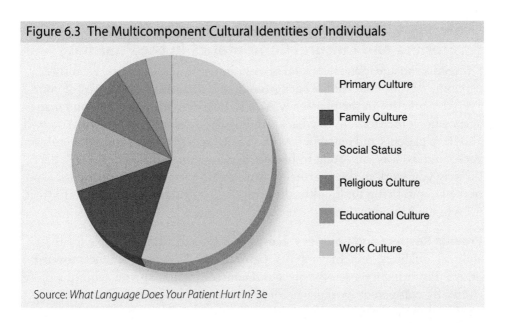

Figure 6.3 The Multicomponent Cultural Identities of Individuals

- Primary Culture
- Family Culture
- Social Status
- Religious Culture
- Educational Culture
- Work Culture

Source: *What Language Does Your Patient Hurt In?* 3e

Individuals are a complex mix, which is why stereotypes are so inaccurate. People are as individualized as their fingerprint. We each have a family of origin with its own history, traditions, and beliefs that exists within a larger community culture, neighborhood, or identity group (such as high school teenagers or seniors). There are layers of socioeconomic status, gender identity, religious identity, politics, educational influences, and work. Figure 6.3 illustrates the various components that make up cultural identity.

When working in the pharmacy, never assume that because someone belongs to an ethnic, racial, or cultural group, that person will necessarily believe or follow the practices generally attributed to that primary group.

Conflict between prescribed medication therapy and a patient's beliefs should be addressed with the prescriber. For example, if an emergency room doctor prescribed a discharge medication for a patient without knowing the specific cultural or religious affiliation, the physician might be unaware of any beliefs or traditions that would influence the types of treatment that the patient may accept or refuse.

Ask questions to better determine the degree of influence that membership in an ethnic, racial, or cultural group has on the individual patient's health—and illness—beliefs and practices. However, proceed with some degree of caution. No one wants to feel interrogated, and many patients may not want to answer personal questions.

Safety Alert

Understanding potential reasons why a patient may not want to fill a prescription may prevent you from asking the wrong questions and accidentally offending the patient. Understanding these reasons will prepare you to offer suggestions of alternative therapies to the patient.

Understanding the Importance of Multicultural Awareness and Cultural Competency in the Pharmacy

Differences in age, gender, sexual orientation, ethnicity, language, culture, economic status, educational background, and disability will be part of your everyday practice in the pharmacy. You will work with coworkers and managers who come from diverse backgrounds different from your own. You will also have patients and customers with various social, ethnic, and other cultural backgrounds. It is important to be aware of how these differences may affect the way you work in the pharmacy, as well as the safety of your patients. One of the keys to being multiculturally aware and culturally competent is to treat everyone with respect and courtesy.

Provide Respect and Courtesy **Respect** means to admire people for their abilities, qualities, or achievements. **Courtesy** is showing politeness toward others. Fostering a sense of respect and courtesy will help you achieve a more culturally competent workplace, for both the patients and customers you serve and the people you work with.

However, there are challenges to behaving respectfully and courteously when dealing with others who have a different background from yours. You may think that you are behaving courteously, but you may accidentally be exhibiting behavior that is seen as disrespectful in a different culture. For example, in most Western countries, maintaining direct eye contact when interacting with others shows that you are paying attention to what they are saying. However, in Asian and Middle Eastern countries, direct eye contact is seen as disrespectful.

Work Wise

Be prepared to modify your cultural norms to accommodate a patient's standards of interactions when possible.

Shaking hands is acceptable and seen as a professional practice in most countries, but some cultures have certain guidelines that differ. For example, using the left hand to shake hands in the Middle East is taboo. Rather than a handshake, in some parts of Europe people greet one another with a kiss in the air near both cheeks.

Being aware and respectful of differences in cultures demonstrates a courtesy to the person and fosters better communication and goodwill. This exemplifies good customer service and carries over to feelings of goodwill for the company you work for.

Consider Safety Failure to consider a patient's cultural identity could lead to safety issues. For example, if you are unable to speak a patient's language, you may not be able to effectively explain a medication, leading to poor adherence by the patient. It may even pose a problem with correctly identifying a patient, which could lead to a misfilled prescription. If patients believe in alternative therapy as part of their cultural traditions, and you are dismissive of these beliefs, they may withhold important information from you and

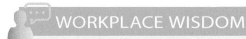
Safety Issues and Language

There are many examples of when a language barrier or cultural misunderstanding can lead to grave safety errors. A patient who spoke only Spanish read a label for methotrexate that was once a week. The only word the patient recognized was "once," which is the number 11 in Spanish. The patient took 11 doses each day and died from an overdose. A patient from Central America had experienced only homeopathic medicine (which says to treat where the issue is). Her daughter had an ear infection and was prescribed tablets to treat it. The mother came to the pharmacy to ask the pharmacist for help because there was no more room for the medicine—she had been placing the tablets into the daughter's ear.

—Anne LaVance, BS, CPhT

other care providers. Some patients may not ask questions about their therapy due to a cultural belief that healthcare providers know what is best, even if that may not always be the case. Some individuals act upon cultural traditions and norms in which women may not be part of decision-making processes related to their care or the care of family members. Caregivers should respect those traditions and norms and interact with a patient's husband, father, or significant other as requested.

According to the American College of Clinical Pharmacy, developing cultural competence in pharmacy practice can increase effectiveness of drug therapy and favorably affect health outcomes.

Understanding Pharmacy Policies

The pharmacy you work for will address diversity issues in your policies and procedures manual. Many pharmacies will also provide you with training on how to be multiculturally aware. Often there is a protocol or procedures to follow when encountering a language barrier, for example.

One of the best ways to promote diversity and awareness of different cultures is for a pharmacy to engage in the predominant demographics that make up its patient base. For example, Walgreens devotes funding and energy toward inclusion of different groups based on location. One of its stores is located in the Castro district of San Francisco, a predominately LGBTQ (lesbian, gay, bisexual, transgender, queer) area of the city. The store worked to include displays and products that celebrated those groups. As a result, the staff was more inclusive—and mutual understanding and acceptance were promoted. In New York, one Walgreens pharmacist addressed the needs of one of its predominant patient populations by working extensively with older HIV-positive patients regarding their therapy.

Safety Alert

When in doubt, ask a pharmacist for assistance. If you think that a language barrier may lead to miscommunication about a medication, telling a pharmacist can help you get the resources you need—whether it is an interpreter, materials printed in another language, or something else to assist the patient.

Another area in which to increase your knowledge and cultural competency is with continuing education courses. Continuing education credits are required for national certification and for many state registrations. These courses typically include written or video materials to review and an assessment. Continuing education is covered further in Module 9.

All workplaces are required to follow antidiscrimination laws. Title VII of the Civil Rights Act of 1964 prohibits discrimination in employment on the basis of race, color, sex, or ethnic origin; the Age Discrimination in the Employment Act prohibits discrimination against employees 40 years of age and older; and the Americans with Disabilities Act prohibits discrimination in employment on the basis of disabilities and requires that employers reasonably accommodate individuals with disabilities who can otherwise perform a job.

6.2 Cultural Considerations in Pharmacy Practice

When you begin your job in a community or institutional pharmacy, you will encounter new cultural scenarios that you have not experienced before. As a student who has chosen to study pharmacy, you may hold certain beliefs regarding the efficacy of Western medications as a preferred treatment for diseases and conditions. However, being culturally aware also means understanding that many patients also hold different beliefs and may be distrustful of doctors and pharmaceutical treatments. To be culturally competent, you need to understand these beliefs and respect those who hold them.

Identifying Cultural Issues Affecting Hispanic Patients

The Hispanic population is growing in the United States, at a rate of 50% since 2000, according to a Pew Research study. Hispanic patients may be more likely to seek treatment at a healthcare clinic located in a pharmacy and value affordable pharmaceuticals.

A large issue you may encounter are patients who speak only Spanish. Having high-quality educational materials printed in both English and Spanish can be very helpful in making your patients feel more comfortable. Having Spanish-speaking pharmacy personnel on staff, or high-quality interpretation mechanisms available, will also assist this patient population.

A factor to consider, especially with Hispanic patients from Mexico who are very new to the United States, is that pharmacies are less regulated in Mexico than in the United States. Mexican laws allow stores to open with only a business license, and pharmacists can work without prior training in dispensing prescriptions. The *farmacia* (pharmacy) in Mexico operates much like an American convenience store, and many medications are available for sale over the counter. Immigrants from Mexico may be unfamiliar with

US regulations regarding controlled substances, refills, etc. Take the time to explain these regulations when possible.

Identifying Cultural Issues Affecting Black and African American Patients

African American and black patients often face discrimination in the healthcare system, which leads to health disparities, including equitable quality of care and access to health care. Economic issues also affect many African American and black patients. Nearly one-third of African Americans do not have a regular doctor, and close to 1.8 million African American children do not have health insurance.

As a pharmacy technician, you can help customers who do not have health insurance seek ways to make their medications more affordable, such as prescription discount programs and asking their providers for generic vs. brand-name drugs when appropriate. It is also important to be empathetic to any economic hardships that you may encounter. By saying something like, "I understand the prices of these medications is high; let me see what options are available that can help lower the cost," you are expressing empathy with the patient's hardship and demonstrating a desire to help. A technician can offer any discount cards or plans that the patient can qualify for to assist them. Sometimes the patient is simply unaware of the options available. Plans and discounts can vary from location to location, so you will need to learn what your setting offers.

Understanding Traditional Chinese Medicine

The history of medicine has roots in several cultures, including ancient Asian (predominantly Chinese), Middle Eastern, European, and African cultures. Traditional Chinese medicine, also sometimes known as *Eastern medicine* or *traditional medicine,* has had a significant influence on most cultures in Asia. Eastern medicine was built on more than 2,500 years of Chinese medical practice, including herbal medicine, acupuncture, massage, and dietary therapy. It is based on the concept of having a balanced qi, energy that flows through the body.

Many aspects of traditional Chinese medicine, including acupuncture/acupressure, herbal medicine, and reflexology, are widely accepted categorically as complementary and alternative medicine by caregivers across the United States. Some services, like acupuncture, are also covered by US health insurance companies.

Western medicine is defined as a system in which doctors and other healthcare professionals treat symptoms and diseases using drugs, radiation, or therapy. It may also be referred to as *conventional medicine* or *mainstream medicine.*

Recognize Alternative Medicine Practices In pharmacy practice, you may encounter those who believe primarily in alternative medicine practices. If patients do not disclose the use of traditional care and remedies to their health-care provider or pharmacist, adverse interactions with prescribed medications are possible. It is important to ask patients if they are taking any medication, including herbal and homeopathic remedies.

Recognize Homeopathy A common alternative therapy you may encounter as a pharmacy technician is homeopathy. **Homeopathy** is a system of alternative medicine created in the 1800s based on the belief that a substance that causes the symptoms of disease in healthy people will cure that disease in sick people. A toxic substance will be greatly diluted (such as one part in 1 trillion) and used to treat illness. For example, Belladonna (a deadly nightshade plant) is diluted and used to treat migraines.

Homeopathy is controversial as some preparations contain substances that may be toxic in humans. In general, the substances are diluted enough that they do not cause adverse effects. However, there have been cases in which the concentration strength of the active ingredient was found to be at toxic levels due to improper dilution. In 2016, the FDA issued a safety alert to consumers warning against the use of homeopathic teething gels and tablets due to the sensitivity of pediatric patients and the fact that these products had not been evaluated or approved by the FDA for safety or efficacy.

> "Many Americans and individuals from other cultures abroad increasingly value complementary and alternative medicine options and have incorporated them into their wellness and preventive medicine practices."

While there are considerations with the use of homeopathy, many Americans and individuals from other cultures abroad increasingly value complementary and alternative medicine options and have incorporated them into their wellness and preventive medicine practices. India has more than 100 million people who practice homeopathy as their primary source of health care. Other countries that include homeopathic remedies in their national health systems are Brazil, Chile, Mexico, Pakistan, Switzerland, and the United Kingdom.

Ask your patients if they are taking homeopathic remedies and respect their answers without judgment. It is crucial to patient safety to understand everything the patient may be taking and how the remedies could interact with their medications.

Think It Through: Customers and Homeopathy

If your pharmacy sells homeopathic remedies, what would you do if a customer came to the pharmacy window and asked your advice about the product?

6.3 Religious Considerations in Pharmacy Practice

In addition to working with colleagues and serving patients of different cultural backgrounds, you will also encounter patients and colleagues who hold religious beliefs that differ from your own. Many religious beliefs, such as Christian Science, Amish, Islam, Christianity, and Jehovah's Witnesses, may have a direct effect on the way you care for your patient. It is important to keep in mind these different beliefs and treat them respectfully.

Many individuals around the world believe there is a link between religion and health and that prayer influences recovery from an illness. Many religions prohibit some treatments and encourage others.

In addition to considering the religious values, beliefs, and traditions of your patients, you also will need to navigate the challenges of working with colleagues who have religious beliefs that are different from your own, and even some that you may not agree with. Some of these beliefs have an effect on the pharmacy operations, such as the recent news stories of pharmacists and pharmacy technicians refusing to dispense prescription contraceptives based on religious or personal beliefs. Pharmacy staff should be aware of their workplace policies related to exercising religious freedom in the performance of the job. It is important to ensure that a company's values do not conflict with yours or require you to do things that may conflict with religious values, beliefs, or traditions.

Work Wise

The key to respectfully communicating with patients and colleagues is to be aware of differences, avoid stereotypes, and practice the communication skills you learned in Module 5.

Identifying Religious Issues Affecting Patients

Working as a pharmacy technician, you may not ever know about your patient's religion, but other times, it may surface as a potential issue or even a barrier to providing patient care. This is not a comprehensive list of existing religious beliefs, merely some examples of the common religions that pharmacy technicians may serve.

Christian Science is a set of beliefs developed in 19th-century New England with the book *Science and Health*. This text argued that sickness is an illusion and can be cured by prayer alone. Therefore, many Christian Science members rely solely on faith healing, and often no medication is given to treat illness. However, the church does not require that Christian Scientists avoid all health care and may make exceptions for services, such as dentistry, optometry, obstetrics, and vaccination, when required by law. It is important not to assume that just because someone is a Christian Scientist that person does not believe in medicine. Respect a Christian Scientist's request to decline some aspects of care.

The Amish religion is known for simple living and the reluctance to adopt technology. Regions with a high Amish population include Pennsylvania, Ohio, Wisconsin, and Indiana. The Amish are open to alternative forms of therapy but are receptive to healthcare information and conventional care when necessary. One consideration when serving Amish customers in the pharmacy is understanding unique English language dialects (Amish individuals speak a dialect called Pennsylvania Dutch or Pennsylvania German, which is a German dialect that often incorporates English words in its everyday usage). There may also be prescription affordability issues, as many Amish customers pay entirely in cash.

Islam is the world's second-largest religion and has over 1.8 billion followers, known as Muslims. In the Islamic religion, many followers believe that physicians have the power to heal, and Muslims believe every illness has a cure and multiple treatment options should be explored. Religious holidays and customs can have an influence on healthcare practices. For Muslims, the month-long fast of Ramadan may interfere with the ability to take prescribed medications on their usual schedules. During this holy month, Muslims do not eat or drink until after sundown.

Christianity is the world's largest religion, with over 2.4 billion followers. There are a multitude of denominations within the Christian faith, each with different traditions and views of the roles of both faith and health care. Because there are so many different branches and denominations of the Christian church, it is important to avoid broad generalizations. Pharmacy technicians should listen to patients' concerns and preferences and respect their decisions related to accepting or declining various forms of health care.

Jehovah's Witness is a religion of around 8.5 million people, headquartered in Warwick, New York. It is against their religious beliefs, values, and traditions to receive blood transfusions. They will accept nonblood alternatives and other medical procedures and treatments. As a pharmacy technician, it is important to be sensitive to the beliefs of a Jehovah's Witness patient and why they may turn down medications in a hospital.

"If you are unaware of a particular belief or practice, open and honest communication with the patient will reveal any issues you need to be aware of."

Because there are so many different religious traditions and practices across our diverse nation, you may feel challenged as a pharmacy technician to provide culturally competent care. However, it is important to know that a universal value across most religious beliefs and practices is to encourage followers to take care of and respect their bodies. While you may not necessarily believe the same things, it can be helpful to keep in mind that most people have the same goal—to live a healthful and happy life. A pharmacy technician should avoid making assumptions about a patient's health based on religious affiliation. Often enough, if you are unaware of a particular belief or practice, open and honest communication with the patient will reveal any issues you need to be aware of.

Identifying Religious Issues Affecting Pharmacy Personnel

Religion is often seen as a topic that most people try to avoid discussing in the workplace. It is often seen as taboo or impolite. However, there are times when a colleague's religion may directly affect the workplace, particularly in a pharmacy.

You may have heard news stories over the last few years detailing pharmacy technicians and pharmacists refusing to fill prescriptions for birth control or sell emergency contraception due to personal or religious beliefs. If a colleague refuses to fill certain prescriptions due to their beliefs, your workload can increase, possibly making you feel resentful.

The laws governing pharmacies vary from state to state, and most states' pharmacy practice acts do not specifically address the issue of refusal to perform a required job task based on personal or religious beliefs. The American Pharmacists Association has issued best practice guidelines that stress the importance of patients having access to legally prescribed medications and a process whereby pharmacies may transfer refused prescriptions to an alternative pharmacy that can fill the patient's prescription. These guidelines place an emphasis on patient care and pharmacies' commitment to meeting customers' needs.

The varying religious traditions, beliefs, and values of pharmacy employees may have an effect on work flow and scheduling as well. Many religious traditions entail holy (special or ceremonial) days that a coworker may have to take off to observe. Your coworker may have to take breaks at certain times during the day for prayer. If lunch is brought in for the pharmacy staff and a coworker doesn't eat it, it may be because of dietary restriction. If you are unsure, an honest and respectful question usually solves this problem.

To effectively navigate various situations with coworkers in the pharmacy, it is important to use the communication tools you learned in Module 5. Avoid placing blame and speak about the issue in a calm tone. Use active listening and speaking skills and restate what you think you heard to the speaker to confirm that you understand what you are being told. Working to understand those with different beliefs is important to a healthy and functioning workplace.

> ### Think It Through: Religious Holidays
> If a coworker was absent due to a religious holiday, how would that make you feel? What would you do if other colleagues were upset or feeling overburdened when another had the day off to observe a religious holiday?

6.4 Gender and Sexuality Considerations in Pharmacy Practice

To understand the complex issues surrounding gender and sexuality and how they relate to your practice in pharmacy, it is first important to understand common terms. **Biological sex** includes the anatomy of an individual's reproductive system and secondary sex characteristics. **Gender** is defined as the range of characteristics pertaining to masculinity and femininity. These characteristics can include biological sex, social structures, such as gender roles, and gender identity. One's **gender identity** refers to personal identification and what pronouns are preferred. Sexual orientation refers to a person's sexual identity in terms of the gender to whom the person is attracted. **LGBTQ** is the acronym used to refer to people who are lesbian (women who are attracted to women), gay (men or women attracted to people of the same gender; more commonly used to describe men), bisexual (people who are attracted to those of the same gender and opposite gender), transgender (those whose gender identity is different from the sex they were assigned at birth), or queer (a term people use to express fluid identities and orientations).

The pharmacy technician should be understanding of the unique health concerns and needs of the LGBTQ populations in the communities they serve. By establishing a comfortable, nonjudgmental environment for the discussion of gender and sexuality issues as they relate to healthcare needs, pharmacy personnel can establish rapport and provide effective treatments for all patients.

Identifying Gender and Sexuality Issues Affecting Patients

Often people prefer to discuss personal medical information with pharmacists or technicians of the same gender. For example, some male customers may feel more comfortable discussing questions on condom use or erectile dysfunction drugs with a male technician or pharmacist. Similar issues may arise in the case of a female customer with issues regarding menstruation or menopause.

You should proceed with caution when addressing patients by a particular pronoun. Some pharmacies and healthcare providers are beginning to ask patients on intake forms which pronoun they prefer. When in doubt, stick to neutral language, such as the singular form of "they," unless corrected. If you make a mistake with a pronoun, a simple apology can help.

Pharmacy technicians should be aware of the history of anti-LGBTQ bias in health care and how that can affect LGBTQ individuals in seeking and receiving culturally competent care. Until 1973, homosexuality was listed as a disorder in the Diagnostic and Statistical Manual of Mental Disorders (DSM), and transgender is still listed in the DSM-5. While attitudes are improving, LGBTQ patients still report reluctance to reveal their sexual orientations or gender identities to their healthcare providers, fearing discrimination or poor treatment. This leads to disparities in the quality and access of appropriate health care for these patients.

LGBTQ people are less likely to have health insurance than heterosexual people, and transgender people have the lowest insurance rates of these groups. As a pharmacy technician, you should be aware of the economic disparity this may cause for these patients and suggest prescription assistance programs they could qualify for.

When serving a transgender patient, you may see that the insurance and identification do not reflect the patient's current name or gender identity. Use caution to make sure you find out the patient's preferred name and use that when filling the prescription.

Transgender patients on hormone therapy are at risk for several complications and side effects. When taking hormones, such as estradiol for gender reassignment, patients are at a higher risk for such diseases as type 2 diabetes, blood clots, cardiovascular disease, and osteoporosis. Smoking enhances these risks, very similar to birth control medications, which also contain hormones. Patients may be reluctant to talk about their medications with the pharmacist, as it would involve discussing their transgender identities. While the transgender community is becoming more accepted, many physicians and caregivers may not be well versed in the nuances of care for this demographic. As a technician communicating with a transgender patient, be sure to suggest talking to the pharmacist regarding therapy, encouraging it as a means to ensure the best care for the patient.

Identifying Gender and Sexuality Issues Affecting Pharmacy Personnel

All pharmacies have antidiscrimination policies stating that employees cannot be discriminated against for their gender or sexual orientation. However, if you encounter or witness discrimination at your workplace, alert a supervisor or the human resources department right away.

If you hear a coworker making a derogatory comment about a patient with regard to the patient's gender or sexual orientation, follow the skills you have learned to be an effective communicator. Clearly and calmly state your position and alert a supervisor about the situation.

> ### Think It Through: Confronting Discrimination
> Have you ever witnessed discrimination, either in the workplace, at school, or in your social life? If so, how did you handle it? Were you a bystander, or did you speak up? What are ways you can speak up if it happens again in the future?

6.5 Culturally Competent Interactions and Communications

There are times when a patient's cultural identity, religious values/beliefs, gender, or sexual orientation may directly or indirectly influence your interactions. Some common issues you may encounter include language issues, differences in the level of eye contact, and titles of address. The same is true for working with pharmacy personnel and other colleagues. The key is to learn about the potential barriers you may encounter; respect others' cultural values, beliefs, and traditions; and work toward effective and empathetic communication that is built upon mutual respect and consideration. To communicate effectively with patients and colleagues of a cultural identity different than your own, it is important to remember the communication skills you learned in Module 5. Using verbal and nonverbal skills, active listening, and speaking skills will assist you in communicating with all patients, regardless of their cultural values, beliefs and traditions, religious background, or gender/sexual identities.

Considering Language Issues

According to the US Census Bureau, English is spoken by 229 million US residents. The next most common language is Spanish, spoken by 40 million US residents, followed by Chinese, spoken by 3 million US residents.

Interpreters are an important part of overcoming language barriers that may affect patients and pharmacy staff members' ability to communicate and interact effectively in the care of the patient. Interpreters should be used

EXPAND YOUR KNOWLEDGE

Family Names in Hispanic Culture

Various dimensions of cultural identity may even affect record keeping. For example, the terms *first name*, *middle name*, and *last name* as used by many Americans (and most pharmacies) cannot be easily used for many Hispanics and Latinos. Many Latinos have as many as four given names (one or more first names and one or more middle name) and two family names. Thus, American healthcare workers can often misunderstand what the true "last" name is,

causing Latinos to be listed multiple times in electronic health record systems or other pharmacy software. As a pharmacy technician, you may need to search in your system for a Latino patient in multiple ways to find the correct record. To learn more about how children are named in Spanish-speaking countries, read the genealogy article at https://SSPharm. ParadigmEducation.com/Genealogy.

to assist patients who speak little to no English, as opposed to deferring that important responsibility to family members or friends. While their intention may be good, family and friends may have low healthcare literacy or could withhold or misinterpret information in translation to the patient. Using family members and friends to interpret could also violate patient confidentiality.

Bilingual pharmacy technicians are always in high demand in the community setting, as they can easily translate for the pharmacist and do not violate HIPAA regulations. When not available, there are subscription-based translation phone services that can be used. To use a translation service, the technician calls the service and identifies the language needed for translation, and then the phone is passed back and forth between the patient and the pharmacy staff, with the translator being the third party. Pharmacies are also more frequently using mobile devices and software, such as Google Translate. In the institutional setting, with its larger staff, a common practice is to have a "translator bank" of various staff members in the facility. The department that needs translation will call the operator, who then identifies those onsite who speak the requested language.

In terms of printed materials, pharmacy database software has the option to print drug monographs and labels in a patient's primary language. The technician chooses the correct language option when entering the patient into the system for the first time, but it may be edited at any time.

WORKPLACE WISDOM

Avoiding Language Assumptions

Being a Hispanic person working in Texas, I have observed a lot of Spanish-speaking customers who come to the pharmacy. I've encountered Spanish speakers who would rather try to speak English than to be humiliated, even if a Spanish speaker is available to translate. They prefer to speak to the person directly rather than having to speak to someone and have them translate. In this case one must be sensitive to the situation. Be sure to remove the customer from an environment filled with other people to prevent distraction. If a translator is needed, explain that to the customer and ask for consent to communicate through a translator. In addition, be sure whoever is translating is actually fluent in the language. Some people get upset if the person translating isn't able to translate properly. Make sure your pharmacy has a trusted method for translating, and also print the instructions in the customer's language.

Also, do not assume that all individuals know how to read. If you ask them, "Do you understand how to read?" they will say yes just to avoid embarrassment. Instead, make sure you point out the important information. All of this can be time consuming, but preventing a medication error is far more important.

—Irene Villatoro, BS, CPhT, RPhT

A common error that individuals make in situations regarding language barriers is to raise the volume of their voice as a means of increasing understanding. This error should be avoided. Do not speak louder when you are speaking to a patient who has limited English-speaking ability. This will not help the patient to hear you better—instead, it may call too much attention to the communication barrier you are facing and embarrass the patient. In fact, some patients may pretend that they understand you rather than admit they are experiencing a language barrier. Instead, approach patients quietly, respecting their right to a confidential conversation, and if necessary, bring in an interpreter to assist.

When communicating with patients who have limited English proficiency, face the patient and make liberal use of common gestures and facial expressions. Observe the patient's face, eyes, and body language carefully, as they may provide clues to help you understand more clearly what they are attempting to communicate. Avoid slang or lingo and speak with as many straightforward terms as possible. Rephrase and restate what you are saying often to confirm understanding between you and the patient. For example, you might rephrase a patient's comment by saying, "You said that you are taking some herbal medicines. What are the names of these herbs?"

Considering Eye Contact Issues

Another area in which cultural traditions and behaviors vary is in the amount of eye contact used during conversations. Americans tend to use direct eye contact and associate it with honesty. Likewise, in some Latin countries, eye contact is important when conveying equality among individuals. However, in some Asian countries, it is considered impolite or disrespectful to establish eye contact with those who hold high positions. Avoiding eye contact is seen as a demonstration of respect.

> "Watch others' behavior and respond accordingly."

To communicate well with your colleagues who may have different cultural norms than yours, make sure you are respectful, and do not make assumptions. Watch others' behavior and respond accordingly. For example, if you are speaking and notice a colleague doesn't hold your gaze, respect that and look away more frequently than you might otherwise.

Considering Titles of Address

People from different cultures may have specific ways of addressing and greeting others, and it can be a challenge to determine how a patient or colleague wishes to be formally addressed. In some cultures, it is inappropriate to address someone by first name.

If you notice that a colleague always addresses you as Mr. Smith, do not continually correct your colleague and insist on being called Joe. Your colleague may hold a cultural belief that requires more formal greetings to be used in the workplace or with superiors. It is appropriate to ask the first time if your colleagues would mind calling you by your first name, but if they continue to use a more formal greeting, let them do so. Also, consider asking them how they prefer to be addressed in the workplace.

Patients may prefer to address you with a formal title because they hold a cultural belief that healthcare personnel should be addressed respectfully and formally. You can ask patients how they prefer to be addressed as you are serving them in the pharmacy. Doing this can also help you navigate serving a transgender patient. Ask patients their preferred names and pronouns to avoid calling them by the wrong pronouns, potentially making them feel poorly about the interaction and your pharmacy.

Communicating with Pharmacy Personnel

Both the National Standards for Culturally and Linguistically appropriate Services (CLAS) and the Joint Commission encourage the continued diversification of healthcare professionals so that their numbers become proportional to the ethnic composition of the communities they serve. A typical pharmacy workplace will continue to diversify, and while this is a positive movement, this diversity of languages and cultures can sometimes pose communication challenges in the workplace.

Various cultural traditions and beliefs inform individuals' ideas concerning the definition of work ethic. In general, **work ethic** may be defined as a set of ideals that drives one's commitment to work hard and produce quality results. How that definition is applied in one's work performance may vary based on an employee's cultural identity. Employees who were raised in an individualistic society, like the United States, may consider self-starting or showing initiative as an ideal demonstration of good work ethic. Conversely, employees who were raised in a collective society, like many Asian nations, may view hard work as being done for the good of all, rather than the individual. Standing out as a harder worker than others could be perceived as causing a superior to "lose face" and might be frowned upon.

Many American workplaces prefer directness in communication style. However, some employees may have been raised with ethnic or family cultural values that dictate that it is impolite to express one's opinion or criticize a colleague. This can pose unique challenges in a pharmacy. As a pharmacy technician, you may find that colleagues have made a mistake and you need to inform them of that mistake. If your colleague's cultural norm says that criticism is considered rude, do your best to frame the problem as an issue to be solved, not something the person has done wrong. Taking a collaborative, team-based approach that focuses on the issue rather than the individual can help soften criticism. There are many tips in Module 5 that can be helpful in difficult situations.

Many pharmacy workplaces provide cultural competence training, or you may take courses on cultural competence in your continuing education throughout your career. Cultural-competence training empowers employees to provide better care to patients from different cultural backgrounds and may also improve communication in the culturally diverse workplace. Improved communication can increase trust among coworkers, improve teamwork, reduce incidents of miscommunication and errors, improve the overall treatment of patients, and increase employees' job satisfaction.

> ### Think It Through: Culture and Misunderstandings
> Perceived rudeness by a colleague may reflect the differences that exist among various cultural values and norms related to social interaction. Consider a time when you may have been misunderstood; how could you have used multicultural awareness to reframe the interaction?

Refrain from Judgment Once you have ascertained how patients' culture influences their healthcare decisions, some culturally competent ways to treat patients and avoid stereotyping include refraining from judgment and honoring a patient's decision-making.

Self-Reflection:
Check How Judgmental You Are

Consider your level of judgment for others. Respond as honestly as possible.
- Do you often judge people for how they dress, speak, or behave?
- How would you rate yourself on a scale of 1 to 5, with 1 being the least judgmental and 5 being the most judgmental? If you rate yourself highly on judgment, consider ways to keep an open mind and honor others' decisions and life choices.

To establish a trusting relationship between a healthcare provider and patient, it is essential to acknowledge the patient's beliefs without criticism. Should a patient disclose use of an intervention or practice that is contraindicative, ask if the patient can speak with the pharmacist about it to ensure proper medication therapy outcomes. Inform the pharmacist of the situation and allow the pharmacist to counsel the patient.

Honor the Patient's Decision-Making Process If the patient's replies to your questions indicate that other people, such as family members, religious leaders, or traditional healers, are involved in the patient's healthcare decisions, it is strongly recommended that these persons be included or acknowledged in any decisions that the patient is being asked to make. Although the American model of health care is based upon the autonomy of patient decisions, this may not be appropriate for patients who view decision-making as a collective endeavor.

Review the Recommended Treatment Plan Patients who view the caregiver or caregiving institution with great deference and authority may appear to agree with treatment plans that they cannot or do not intend to follow. This is because they feel it is more polite to pretend to agree rather than to argue with authority. Therefore, when reviewing a patient's medications that may require following a daily diet plan or changing activities, ascertain the patient's typical diet and daily habits. With this knowledge, ask the pharmacist to make suggestions for possible alternatives that may work better for the patient, without criticizing the patient's present habits.

6.6 Module Summary

As a pharmacy technician, your goal should be to provide culturally competent care to all patients—regardless of their race, ethnicity, gender, sexual orientation, or any other group with whom they identify. The key is to keep an open mind and learn more about people's beliefs, cultural traditions and values, and life experiences and to treat them with respect. Keep in mind that you may make mistakes, but if you put your patient's satisfaction, dignity, and right to receive quality care above all else, that commitment will positively influence how you interact with them. Patients who sense empathy on the part of their caregivers will feel safe and open to helping you learn how they would like to be treated in your pharmacy. Being receptive, tolerant, and respectful of other beliefs is the foundation of cultural competency.

 The online course includes additional review and assessment resources.

Law & Ethics

LEARNING OBJECTIVES

1 Understand the differences between state and federal laws and regulations. (Section 7.1)

2 Learn the influence of state and federal regulatory agencies on pharmacy practice. (Section 7.1)

3 Identify legal requirements for pharmacy technicians to practice. (Section 7.2)

4 Identify federal laws and regulations related to drug manufacturing. (Section 7.3)

5 Identify federal laws and regulations related to drug packaging. (Section 7.4)

6 Identify federal laws and regulations related to drug labeling, marketing, and advertising. (Section 7.5)

7 Identify federal laws and regulations related to compounding. (Section 7.6)

8 Identify federal laws and regulations related to dispensing. (Section 7.7)

9 Identify federal laws and regulations related to medication safety. (Section 7.8)

10 Identify federal laws and regulations related to insurance. (Section 7.9)

11 Understand professional practice standards. (Section 7.10)

12 Use codes of conduct and ethical standards in practice. (Section 7.11)

P harmacy technician students learn the federal laws and regulations that govern pharmacy practice. These laws and regulations, coupled with state board of pharmacy regulations, lay the foundation for a facility's policies and procedures as well as guide your professional communications and behaviors with colleagues and patients. Therefore, your knowledge of federal and state legislation and its application to pharmacy practice is critical to fulfilling your work responsibilities.

You must also learn federal laws and regulations to sit for a national certification exam for pharmacy technicians. The Pharmacy Technician Certification Exam (PTCE) and the Exam for the Certification of Pharmacy Technicians (ExCPT) contain questions that assess your knowledge of pharmacy law and its application in the field. According to the blueprints for each exam, the PTCE devotes 12.5% of its exam to the pharmacy law knowledge area, and the ExCPT allocates 35% of its exam. Remember that these test questions are related to federal laws and regulations that apply to all of the US and its territories. State-specific laws and regulations can vary.

This module provides an overview of key legislation that affects your daily pharmacy practice. You will review the federal rules and regulations, including why they were created and how they influence pharmacy operations. You will also learn the relationship between pharmacy laws and ethical decision-making and behaviors in the practice setting.

Practice Tip

When a conflict exists between a state law and a federal law, the more stringent of the two laws always applies.

7.1 Governmental Oversight of Pharmacy Practice

As mentioned earlier, both US federal and state legislatures create laws and regulations for pharmacy practice. These laws and regulations ensure the safety and well-being of US citizens, which is one of the key responsibilities of our government. Federal laws dictate everything from patient confidentiality to dispensing practices to drug manufacturing guidelines. Consequently, it is important to remember the events that precipitated the establishment of these laws and the impact on facilities, pharmacy personnel, and patients if not adhering to these regulations.

Understanding Federal Laws and Regulations

A **law** is a rule established by an authority to direct behavior. Federal laws govern the practice and operation of pharmacies and the creation and use of medications in the US. A **regulation** is a rule created to enforce a given law. Federal regulations provide the structure and guidance for pharmacy personnel to follow these laws.

Recognize Federal Laws Related to Pharmacy Practice Federal laws typically offer a *minimum level of acceptable standards* as they apply to pharmacy practice. The common mandate of federal laws is the protection of the public. This consumer protection, however, was not always in place. Before the start of the 20th century, the unregulated production and dispensing of medications led to health risks, injuries, and deaths. These events sparked the enactment of federal laws and regulations during the 20th century that addressed the safe manufacturing, labeling, distribution, storage, dispensing, and administration of medications. Today, the US federal laws related to pharmacy practice are some of the strictest regulations in the world. These tight drug controls have safeguarded the health of US citizens for more than a century. For a timeline of federal healthcare legislation and the impact of these laws on pharmacy practice, refer to Table 7.1.

Table 7.1 Significant Federal Healthcare Legislation

Legislation	Impacts on Pharmacy Practice
Pure Food and Drug Act of 1906	created standards for medication ingredients and labeling
Food, Drug, and Cosmetic Act of 1938	established the US Food and Drug Administration (FDA) and enforceable safety standards for medications
Durham Humphrey Amendment of 1951	created legend and over-the-counter classifications for medications; also created standards for the receipt and refill of prescriptions
Controlled Substances Act of 1970	established the Drug Enforcement Administration (DEA), which set regulations for addictive substances
Poison Prevention Packaging Act of 1970	set standards and requirements for childproof packaging of medications
Drug Listing Act of 1972	created national drug codes for medications
Omnibus Budget Reconciliation Act of 1990 (OBRA '90)	required a drug utilization review board and medication history
Dietary Supplement Health and Education Act of 1994	increased FDA oversight and regulation of dietary supplements
Health Insurance Portability and Accountability Act (HIPAA) of 1996	established requirements for the security and privacy of patient health information
FDA Modernization Act of 1997	implemented small-batch pharmacy compounding protocols; shortened legend on prescription medications to "Rx Only"
Medicare Prescription Drug, Improvement, and Modernization Act (MMA) of 2003	created Medicare Part D insurance coverage for prescriptions
Combat Methamphetamine Epidemic Act of 2005	placed controls on sales of pseudoephedrine-containing over-the-counter medications

Recognize the Impact of Federal Regulatory Agencies To provide oversight and enforcement of federal laws and regulations, the US government has established federal regulatory agencies. For example, the Centers for Medicare & Medicaid Services is a federal regulatory agency that implements the Medicare Prescription Drug, Improvement, and Modernization Act of 2003. This agency, as well as other agencies related to pharmacy practice, are listed in Table 7.2.

Table 7.2 Federal Regulatory Agencies Related to Pharmacy Practice

Federal Regulatory Agency	Role and Responsibilities
Centers for Medicaid & Medicare Services	• administers the Medicare program • works with state governments to administer Medicaid • establishes pricing data that is instrumental for the business operations of a pharmacy, such as insurance reimbursement
Drug Enforcement Administration	• is the primary agency responsible for enforcing the laws regarding illegal trafficking of drugs • supervises the legal and illegal use of narcotics and other controlled substances • issues licenses to medical practitioners to write prescriptions for scheduled drugs and to individual pharmacies to order scheduled drugs from wholesalers
Federal Trade Commission	• protects the US consumer from deceptive advertising practices in the marketplace • regulates the labeling and advertising claims of dietary supplements
Food and Drug Administration	• is part of the US Department of Health and Human Services • provides regulations on the drug approval process, generic drug substitution, patient counseling, and adverse reaction reporting systems • issues drug recalls • enforces packaging, labeling, advertising, and marketing guidelines for medications
Occupational Safety and Health Administration	• is an agency of the US Department of Labor • enforces the Bloodborne Pathogens Standard, which prescribes safeguards to protect workers against the health hazards caused by bloodborne pathogens • enforces the Hazard Communication Standard, which ensures that the hazards associated with US manufactured or imported chemicals are evaluated and then communicated to healthcare personnel • ensures the safety and health of US workers by setting and enforcing regulations and standards • provides training, outreach, and education • establishes partnerships • encourages continual improvement in workplace safety and health • investigates any personnel complaints about the safety of a work environment

Understanding State Laws and Regulations Related to Pharmacy Practice

Similar to the federal government, a state's House of Representatives and Senate pass legislation and rely on regulatory agencies to oversee and enforce laws and regulations within the state. State laws and regulations focus on specific aspects of pharmacy practice, such as distribution and administration of medications, the ratio of pharmacists to technicians that can practice in a setting, and so on.

Recognize State Laws Related to Pharmacy Practice Laws and their regulations relating to pharmacy practice differ from state to state. Many of these laws deal specifically with pharmacy technicians, including their education, registration or licensure, national certification requirements, and scope of practice.

For example, the laws in North Carolina for technician registration state that an applicant must do the following:

- hold a high school diploma or equivalent or is currently enrolled in a program that awards a high school diploma
- be employed by a pharmacy holding a valid in-state pharmacy permit
- complete a training program approved by the supervising pharmacist-manager that includes pharmacy terminology, pharmacy calculations, dispensing systems and labeling requirements, pharmacy laws and regulations, record keeping and documentation, and the proper handling and storage of medications, or;
- hold a current pharmacy technician certification issued by the Pharmacy Technician Certification Board (PTCB)

Whereas, in Arizona, to register as a technician, one must do the following:

- have proof of legal residency and birth date
- have a government-issued photo ID
- provide proof of passing the PTCB or ExCPT exam
- obtain a copy of a valid Arizona fingerprint clearance card

While North Carolina has the option of being nationally certified, it is not mandatory, and there is an alternate route to licensure. Arizona, on the other hand, requires national certification as a prerequisite. While there are some similarities in many states, there are also clear differences regarding the laws governing many aspects of pharmacy practice. This difference is due to the composition of members of both the state boards and their respective state legislatures. These members can advocate for new regulations and laws, or they can advocate to not add new requirements or rules.

The Importance of Regulations

Before 2006, Ohio did not have any regulations regarding the training of pharmacy technicians. One could apply for a position without any experience. Unfortunately, this lack of oversight came at a human cost: a tragic medication error made by a pharmacy technician.

In 2006, two-year-old Emily Jerry was receiving intravenous (IV) chemotherapy for an abdominal tumor. During her final chemotherapy treatment, she received a fatal dose of sodium chloride in her IV bag. A pharmacy technician made a medication error when preparing her IV solution.

To find a purpose for his daughter's death, Christopher Jerry established the Emily Jerry Foundation to raise awareness of medication errors and to ensure that pharmacy technicians receive proper education and training to practice. Part of the organization's initiative is to create public awareness of the variation in state laws and regulations governing pharmacy technician practice. To that end, the Emily Jerry Foundation, in cooperation with the American Society of Health-System Pharmacists, created an interactive map to show how your state's pharmacy technicians compare with other states in education and training, certification, registration and licensure, and continuing education. This map can be accessed at **https://SSPharm.ParadigmEducation.com/EmilyJerry**.

Practice Tip

If a regulation or law is being intentionally broken by your pharmacy and you cannot report it internally, you have the option to report the violation to your state BOP. This report can be anonymous if you fear retribution.

Recognize the Impact of State Regulatory Agencies Regulations for pharmacy practice at the state level are established and enforced by that state's board of pharmacy (BOP). To review a summary of the roles and responsibilities of a state's BOP, refer to Table 7.3. Inspectors who work for a state's BOP visit pharmacies to ensure that regulations are being followed by a practice site as well as by pharmacy personnel. These inspections are typically conducted on an annual basis but can be initiated by a complaint or request, either from the public or an employee. For example, Nevada has a regulation that a pharmacy must have a ratio of three pharmacy technicians to one pharmacist (3:1) during hours of operation. If an inspector were to enter a pharmacy where this ratio was not being followed, it would be a finding and potential citation. Other states have different ratios, and some have no ratios. The website for a state's BOP provides information on the state laws and regulations for pharmacy practice as well as the requirements for pharmacy technicians to work in that state. These laws and regulations should be reviewed before moving to a new state to work as a pharmacy technician. A breakdown of BOP roles is outlined in Table 7.3.

Table 7.3 Board of Pharmacy Roles

State Regulatory Agency	Roles and Responsibilities
Board of Pharmacy	• is composed of governor-appointed leaders from the pharmacy community as well as consumer representatives • regulates pharmacists and pharmacy technicians within that state • works with the state's Department of Health • advises state legislators on pharmacy laws and regulations • oversees the inspections of new pharmacies • establishes the required education and training of pharmacists and pharmacy technicians, age requirements, background checks, etc. • maintains a database of all active pharmacist licenses and pharmacy technician licenses (if required by the state), the annual registration of pharmacy technicians, and any certifications • may set the legal pharmacist-to-pharmacy technician ratio • licenses the operation of pharmacies within the state • conducts unannounced inspections to ensure that facilities are complying with the regulations of the Department of Health

7.2 Federal and State Laws Related to Pharmacy Personnel

The overarching purpose of federal and state pharmacy laws is to promote patient safety. These laws address several **practice domains**, including who can dispense medications, what requirements these individuals must fulfill, and what duties these workers can perform.

As mentioned earlier in this module, it is your responsibility to know the legal requirements for pharmacy technicians in your state of practice. These requirements address the licensure, registration, and/or certification of technicians as well as their scope of practice.

Achieving Licensure, Certification, and Registration

The terms *licensure* and *registration* are often used interchangeably when discussing pharmacy technician practice, but these terms reflect different processes with distinct requirements. **Licensure** requires you to take a state exam and meet or exceed a predetermined passing rate, much like taking a state driver's test to be licensed to drive a car. **Certification** requires you to pass a national exam, such as the PTCE or ExCPT. **Registration** requires you to meet state requirements to be placed on a registry or list of pharmacy technicians. These state requirements may include passing a national certification exam, completing an approved training program, or fulfilling a certain number of on-the-job training hours. According to the National Association of Boards of Pharmacy, 12 states license pharmacy technicians, 34 states register technicians, and 21 states require technicians to earn national certification.

Knowing the Scope of Practice

At its core, a pharmacy technician's scope of practice is to assist the pharmacist with the preparation (selection, counting, and packaging) of medications and their subsequent dispensing to patients. How much a technician can assist and in what ways varies among states. For example, in Utah, a pharmacy technician (under the direction of the supervising pharmacist) may advise patients regarding over-the-counter (OTC) medications and dietary supplements. In Maryland, however, pharmacy technicians may *not* advise patients regarding OTC medications. One task that exceeds the scope of practice for pharmacy technicians in all states is offering advice or counsel to patients regarding their prescription medications. This task requires the professional expertise of a pharmacist.

"One task that exceeds the scope of practice for pharmacy technicians in all states is offering advice or counsel to patients regarding their prescription medications."

The scope of practice for pharmacists continues to evolve, which affects the scope of practice for pharmacy technicians. New duties and responsibilities that do not require the professional judgment of a pharmacist are being delegated to technicians in some states. For that reason, you must know the laws and regulations regarding pharmacy technicians in the state in which you practice.

WORKPLACE WISDOM

A Technician's Role in Vaccination

In 2017, Idaho drafted new legislation that allowed certified pharmacy technicians to administer immunization injections under the supervision of a pharmacist. This expanded scope of practice is an exciting glimpse into the future of the pharmacy technician profession. To learn more about the role of pharmacy technicians in Idaho's pharmacy vaccination program, refer to the *Pharmacy Times* article at https://SSPharm.ParadigmEducation.com/Vaccines.

7.3 Federal Laws and Regulations Related to Drug Manufacturing

Before the start of the 20th century, there were no US laws that governed the production and sale of medications. Many people and companies sold counterfeit, adulterated, and in some cases toxic chemicals for consumers to ingest. The snake oil salesmen who would come to a town and sell their magical "cure-all tonic" (which was mainly whiskey) is an example of this type of practice.

The Pure Food and Drug Act of 1906 defined the terms *adulterated* and *misbranded*, which made it a criminal act for businesses to make false claims on their packaging and not listing their ingredients properly. It was a start for drug regulation but required further legislation for it to be enforced.

The federal laws and regulations that helped promote safe drug manufacturing include the FD&C Act of 1938, the Kefauver-Harris Amendment, and the Dietary Supplement Health and Education Act of 1994.

Understanding the Food, Drug, and Cosmetic (FD&C) Act of 1938

The federal Food, Drug, and Cosmetic (FD&C) Act of 1938 was a set of laws crafted to oversee the safety of food, drugs, medical devices, and cosmetics. Cosmetics were added because there were many instances of unsafe products that were causing harm to consumers just as severe as misbranded or adulterated food and drugs. It defined what constitutes food, drugs and devices, or cosmetics and established both civil and criminal penalties for violations. It also established the FDA as an agency that would enforce manufacturing and advertising regulations in the US. The FDA requires that pharmaceutical manufacturers obtain approval before the release of a new drug. This federal law also set quality standards for food, drugs, medical devices, and cosmetics manufactured and sold in the United States. This act is referenced in several areas of this module, as its laws apply to many areas of pharmacy practice.

The FD&C Act and FDA as an agency are two of the reasons that medications are as safe and effective as they are currently. There have also been several amendments to the FD&C Act that have expanded its scope and further defined how pharmacy is practiced.

The FD&C Act of 1938 also set standards for quality ingredients for medications. These standards included drug strength, quality, and purity. This act is where the phrase and standard "pharmacy grade" came to be used, which describes a substance that meets a high level of purity and quality. If a drug, food, or cosmetic is not certified by the FDA, its contents or purity are in doubt and not considered safe for use or consumption. If an approved substance falls into this category, the FDA has the authority to recall it from the US market.

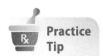

Understanding the Kefauver-Harris Amendment

The Kefauver-Harris Amendment of 1962 was an amendment to the FD&C Act. It requires that the manufacturer of any new drug provide evidence of its safety and effectiveness before the drug can enter the US market. The drug must be shown to be safe through an intensive testing process that is undertaken by a drug sponsor, which is usually a pharmaceutical company. A drug sponsor must obtain permission from the FDA before testing any new drugs. The FDA also requires a pharmaceutical manufacturer to file a new drug application (NDA) with each new drug and to undergo drug trials to obtain FDA approval before marketing. These drug trials take more than a year to complete and involve animal testing and human clinical studies.

The lengthy and rigorous drug trial process is the reason that brand medications are so expensive. The company that paid millions of dollars for years of clinical testing is granted a right to sell the medication exclusively for a period, and the higher consumer cost helps to recoup those research costs. These drug trials also determine the possible side effects of the medication, which is the information that goes into the marketing and patient monographs printed and dispensed with the medication.

Understanding the Dietary Supplement Health and Education Act of 1994

The Dietary Supplement Health and Education Act of 1994 provides guidelines on dietary supplements, including vitamins, minerals, herbs, and nutritional supplements. This legislation states that manufacturers of supplements are *not required* to provide proof of efficacy or standardization to the FDA. Manufacturers simply must prove consumer safety and make truthful claims about their product. Due to the requirements of this act, the language on packaging and marketing materials for these supplements cannot make any claims that they treat a specific disease or condition, as they do not undergo the rigorous testing that drug manufacturers who apply for an NDA do.

"Pharmacy personnel must be prepared to explain how dietary supplement regulation differs from other OTC drugs."

Pharmacy personnel must be prepared to explain how dietary supplement regulation differs from other OTC drugs. Many patients do not understand this distinction and treat vitamins and supplements as if they were FDA-approved medications. These products are not held to the same standards as medications and may vary in quality and potency. It is important for pharmacy technicians to help identify if a patient is taking supplements, as they can interact with prescribed medications.

7.4 Federal Laws and Regulations Related to Drug Packaging

After laws were created regulating the manufacturing of medications themselves, further legislation was needed to govern the way medications were packaged. Until 1970, there were numerous instances of children poisoning themselves by ingesting or being exposed to household substances and chemicals. Pediatricians considered this to be the leading cause of injuries for children under five years of age. The Poison and Prevention Packaging Act of 1970 was enacted to reduce these injuries and fatalities.

Understanding the Poison and Prevention Packaging Act of 1970

The Poison and Prevention Packaging Act required most OTC and prescription drugs to be packaged in child-resistant containers to prevent accidental ingestion by children. To qualify as child resistant, the packaging cannot be opened by 80% of children under age five but can be opened by 90% of adults in manufacturers' tests.

This federal legislation dictates that pharmacy personnel must dispense all prescription medications, including investigational drugs, in child-resistant containers, unless a patient specifically requests a regular container. Many pharmacies include in their new patient intake form a question asking if they would like to opt out of the child-resistant container requirement. This section asks if patients want medication dispensed with "EZ open" lids. If they choose to opt out, the technician has them sign a written or electronic waiver for documentation purposes.

Unit-dose packaging, including blister packs and pouches, must also be child resistant. An extra layer of backing on these medications must be peeled away before the medication can be accessed.

Understanding Additional Considerations Related to Drug Packaging

A drug's packaging plays an important role in its safety and effectiveness. Packaging protects the drug from being exposed to the elements and being contaminated. FDA regulations state that pharmaceutical packaging should provide certain consumer protections. For example, the FDA provides regulations that drug packaging must provide protection against light, moisture, and temperature variations, all of which can change a medication's quality.

FDA regulations also state that drugs should be protected against damage during shipping, handling, and storage. The containers themselves should not interact with a medications' properties or allow leaks.

Safety Alert

Many brands of prescription vials have reversible lids. One side has a childproof locking mechanism, but when flipped, the lid becomes an easy-to-open screw top. Be aware of packaging preferences for each patient. To be packaged with the easy-open mechanism, a patient must request it and, in some cases, sign a waiver.

7.5 Federal Laws and Regulations Related to Drug Labeling, Advertising, and Marketing

In addition to regulating who can practice pharmacy and how drugs must be manufactured and packaged, laws and regulations define how medications must be labeled and advertised to patients and consumers. We often see advertisements on television for new medications and look at medication instructions before using them but may not realize the rules that govern their content.

Federal laws and regulations relating to labeling, advertising, and marketing include the FD&C Act of 1938, the Durham-Humphrey Amendment of 1951, and the Drug Listing Act of 1972.

Understanding the FD&C Act of 1938 as it Relates to Drug Labeling, Advertising, and Marketing

In addition to manufacturing practices, the FDA must oversee the labeling, advertising, and marketing of pharmaceutical products by their manufacturers. For example, manufacturers may not make speculative or false claims about the potential of the product, and they must also disclose the side effects, adverse reactions, and contraindications for their manufactured medications. OTC medications also undergo scrutiny by the FDA. The labels of OTC products must conform to a preferred format to make all information understandable to the public.

While pharmacy technicians are never allowed to provide counseling, identification of existing information on labels both for prescription and OTC medications is legal, as it is considered a statement of fact rather than a professional judgment. If patients cannot read the label, a technician is able to tell them what it says. The FD&C label requirements for OTC medications ensures that accurate information is available to the consumer.

EXPAND YOUR KNOWLEDGE

Problematic Drug Ads

The drug manufacturer Pfizer paid royalties to Queen for the use of the song "We Are the Champions" in one of its advertisements for Viagra. The ad can be viewed at https://SSPharm.ParadigmEducation.com/Viagra.

Did you notice that it was missing certain FDA-required elements in its marketing? The only thing stated at the end was for patients to "talk to their doctor." This ad was pulled from US markets because it did not list the medication's side effects.

Understanding the Durham-Humphrey Amendment of 1951

The Durham-Humphrey Amendment of 1951 established the terms *legend* (prescription required) and *over the counter* regarding medications. The amendment also created provisions that allowed for prescriptions to have refills and for prescribers to be able to call in prescriptions and refills via telephone. Before this, prescriptions had to be handwritten and delivered in person to the pharmacy to be filled.

The Durham-Humphrey Amendment is why labeling on all prescription medications says "Rx Only." These are the medications that must be stored behind the counter. The amendment also set the standards of what drugs can be sold over the counter. It required review by the FDA to determine if a substance could be used safely and effectively without the patient being under the care of a physician.

The labeling requirements for each class are different, with OTC medications having all the required storage and dosing information printed on the bottle or included in the packaging. This information is like the monographs dispensed with prescription medications. The labels or packages must include possible side effects, precautions, dosing ranges, and instructions for use by the patient.

Safety Alert

A pharmacy may have stock bottles of OTC medications, such as Claritin or Benadryl, behind the counter for prescription dispensing. These bottles do not have the FDA-required information printed on them and cannot be sold in the stock bottles as an OTC. The medication must be transferred to a pill vial, which does have the required information from the label generated by the pharmacy software.

Understanding the Drug Listing Act of 1972

The Drug Listing Act of 1972 gave the FDA the authority to compile a list of currently marketed drugs and assign them each a numbered code, called the *national drug code (NDC) number.* That way, the FDA can maintain a database of drugs by use, manufacturer, and active ingredients. With different medications that could have potential allergies, interactions, duplication of therapy, and contraindications, this list is an invaluable resource to healthcare professionals and patients alike.

The NDC number is a unique 10-digit, 3-segment number that is present on all OTC drugs and prescription medication packages and inserts in the United States. The three segments identify the labeler (manufacturer, repackaged, or distributor), the product (specific strength, dosage form, and formulation), and the size and type of its packaging. The NDC number is one of the primary means technicians use to select the proper medication for dispensing, avoid medication errors, and bill insurance. Figure 7.1 illustrates an example of an NDC number.

Figure 7.1 NDC Number

Example: Care One ibuprofen 200 mg has the following NDC number:

Manufacturer	Product code	Package code

$$41520 - 647 - 78$$

41520 identifies the manufacturer, S&S Brands, LLC. All products from this manufacturer begin with this number.

647 identifies the drug as ibuprofen 200 mg.

78 identifies the package size—in this case, 100 caplets. A bottle of 50 caplets would have a different number here.

For billing purposes, the NDC number shows the insurance carrier exactly which medication was dispensed to the customer. For that reason, it is important that the NDC number submitted for payment corresponds with the NDC number of the product actually dispensed. While two different manufacturers may have the exact same medication that would be therapeutically equivalent, they may not be billed the same.

7.6 Federal Laws and Regulations Related to Pharmacy Compounding

Compounding was a fundamental component of the origin of pharmacy practice. From apothecaries to early pharmacy practice, the art and science of mixing compounds for medicinal purposes was the main method for dispensing medications. The advent of large manufacturers and mass-produced medications in the first half of the 20th century became the primary means of medication production. Compounding by pharmacy personnel became the exception rather than the norm.

However, the practice of both sterile and nonsterile compounding is still practiced, and custom preparations are still prescribed and used today. Sterile compounding is a mainstay of hospital practice and numerous specialty pharmacies compound medications for their patients. There is still a need for specific doses of medication that are not available commercially. For nonsterile preparations, these can include hormone therapies, flavor modifications, and dose form changes. Sterile preparations, such as IVs, are by nature customized to modify doses when a patient is in the hospital. Weight-based doses and items, such as total parenteral nutrition, require a technician to compound daily.

Federal laws and regulations related to pharmacy compounding include the FDA Modernization Act of 1997 and the *United States Pharmacopeia (USP)* Chapter <795>, <797>, and <800> Regulations.

Understanding the FDA Modernization Act of 1997

The **United States Pharmacopeia (USP)** is a compendium of drug information for the US that establishes the standards of quality and safety for medications for the entire country. The FDA Modernization Act is an amendment to the FD&C Act that allows pharmacy personnel to compound sterile and nonsterile medications for patients if these medications meet USP standards. A pharmacy that compounds medications for patient-specific doses is different from a manufacturer, such as GlaxoSmithKline, which compounds non–patient-specific medications in bulk for sale. The FDA Modernization Act sets a clear definition of what activities are reserved for each entity, which helps prevent a compounding pharmacy from straying into the realm of manufacturing.

Compounding pharmacies and hospitals do not have to meet the same guidelines as those set for manufacturers. These pharmacies and hospitals mix existing medications into alternate dosages and dose forms for patient-specific prescriptions and orders but do not produce new or unique substances. While small batches can be made in anticipation of use by certain patients, these preparations are not mass produced, which would cross the legal boundary into manufacturing. Manufacturers have stricter guidelines on the sterility and production processes than a compounding pharmacy does.

EXPAND YOUR KNOWLEDGE

Unsafe Compounding Practices

In 2012, there was an outbreak of fungal meningitis that led to the deaths of 76 patients. The outbreak was the result of contaminated compounded preparations from a compounding pharmacy in New England. The pharmacy was making batches of prednisolone epidural injections in bulk rather than patient-specific doses by prescription. The pharmacy was acting like a manufacturer, which broke the laws that regulate compounding pharmacies. The pharmacy was also compounding under unsanitary conditions and falsifying documentation. The 2012 outbreak led to stronger FDA oversight of compounding practices across the country. More information can be found at https://SSPharm.ParadigmEducation.com/FDA.

Understanding *USP* Chapter <795>, <797>, and <800> Regulations

The USP is not a federal or state regulatory agency but is run by a nonprofit organization. USP works closely with government and regulatory agencies to set medication standards. More than 1,000 general chapters in the *USP* cover standards regarding strength, quality, and purity of all drugs and supplements used in the US. These standards are legally recognized in the US. Many of the *USP* chapters apply to manufacturers and distribution, but three are directly related to compounding in pharmacies. These chapters relate to nonsterile compounding (*USP* Chapter <795>), sterile compounding (*USP* Chapter <797>), and hazardous compounding (*USP* Chapter <800>).

The design and maintenance of compounding areas, procedures of compounding personnel, and documentation protocols are covered in *USP* Chapters <795>, <797>, and <800>, depending on the type of compounding involved. This module seeks to highlight key outcomes and practices as a result of these regulations.

Recognize *USP* Chapter <795> *USP* Chapter <795> covers the policies and procedures for nonsterile compounding. Nonsterile compounding includes preparations such as ointments, creams, oral suspensions, and capsules.

Some pharmacy practices that are a result of *USP* Chapter <795> include the following:

- standards for expiration dates of compounded preparations (beyond use dating)
- standardized recipes and procedures for compounded preparations in a master formulation record
- continuing education requirements for compounding personnel to maintain competency in nonsterile compounding

Recognize *USP* Chapter <797> (Rev. 2019) *USP* Chapter <797> (rev. 2019) covers the policies and procedures for sterile compounding—preparations such as standard IV medications and ocular preparations. Compounded sterile preparations (CSPs), are typically large-volume IV solutions used for fluid replacement, small-volume preparations containing an antibiotic in a base solution, narcotic preparations for pain relief, total parenteral nutrition, or chemotherapy medications. Ocular preparations are rarer CSPs prepared by personnel. Because these medications are typically administered by IV or IM routes (less by ocular instillation), the drugs have systemic access via a patient's bloodstream and, consequently, circulate to all organs. For that reason, any breach in aseptic technique during the preparation of a CSP has the potential to contaminate the CSP. This contamination can lead to patient injury or death. Once a contaminated CSP is in a patient's bloodstream, it cannot be reversed. As a result, the guidelines for CSPs are very strict and use highly specialized equipment and environments.

Some pharmacy practices that are a result of *USP* Chapter <797> (rev. 2019) include the following:

- design characteristics of two types of sterile compounding environments: cleanroom suite (ante-room and buffer room) and segregated compounding area
- quality assurance procedures for sterile compounding environments: air quality, temperature, and humidity; microbial air and surface sampling
- equipment used for the preparation of CSPs (laminar airflow systems in primary engineering controls, or hoods)
- CSP quality assurance (risk categories, beyond-use dates, identification of sources of contamination)
- sterile compounding personnel compliance with hand hygiene, garbing, cleaning and disinfection in ante-room and buffer room

Recognize *USP* Chapter <800> *USP* Chapter <800> covers the policies and procedures for compounding of hazardous drugs. These preparations can be harmful to the person preparing them. They can include chemotherapeutic agents, hormone preparations, or radiopharmaceuticals. Because of the risk factors involved, additional precautions and practices are outlined in *USP* <800>.

Some pharmacy practices that are a result of *USP* Chapter <800> include the following:

- design characteristics of a hazardous drug compounding environment: negative-pressure primary engineering control (Class I through Class III biological safety cabinets) in a negative-pressure room
- quality assurance procedures for hazardous drug compounding environment: air quality, temperature, and humidity; microbial air and surface sampling
- identification of hazardous drugs, their associated hazards, safe handling practices, spill management, storage, transport, and disposal
- specific garbing standards for sterile compounding personnel: chemotherapy gown, second pair of shoe covers, chemotherapy gloves, eye and face protection
- specialized equipment for handling hazardous drugs: plastic-backed preparation mat, closed-system transfer device, chemotherapy dispensing pin, and chemotherapy sharps container

7.7 Federal Laws and Regulations Related to Pharmacy Dispensing

Federal laws and regulations pertaining to dispensing are some of the most relevant to pharmacy technicians, especially in the community setting. The main duty of a technician is to assist in the dispensing of medications, whether that entails completing a new patient intake, entering a prescription, preparing an order, or accepting payment. The Controlled Substances Act and OBRA further specified dispensing operations for pharmacy personnel. These acts delineated which medications technicians could handle for production, established protocols for entering controlled substance prescriptions, and created duties related to medication therapy management. Another important act related to dispensing is the Health Insurance Portability and Accountability Act (HIPAA) of 1996.

Understanding the Controlled Substances Act

The Controlled Substances Act of 1970 was created to combat and control drug abuse. This legislation classifies drugs that have the potential for abuse and dependence into schedules, based on their abuse potential. Schedule I (CI) substances are illegal and available only for research or experimental purposes. Schedule II–V (CII–CV) substances can be legally dispensed, with restrictions on the numbers of refills and their quantities. CII medications have the highest potential for abuse, while CV medications have the least. Examples of CII medications include hydrocodone, Ritalin, and morphine. Anabolic steroids and buprenorphine are examples of CIII medications. CIV medications include Valium, Soma, and Xanax. Medications in the CV class include Phenergan with codeine. According to different state regulations, various medications can be treated in the same manner as CV drugs even if they are not officially classified as such, such as pseudoephedrine.

Much like the FD&C Act created the FDA, the Controlled Substances Act created the Drug Enforcement Administration (DEA), whose purpose is to enforce the laws and regulations specifically dealing with controlled substances.

Because of the potential for abuse, the inventory and dispensing procedures for controlled substances are strictly regulated. As a technician, it is important to know which medications and medication classes fall into these categories. If you do not know that a medication is a CII, for example, you might be looking for it on the regular stock shelf when it would, in fact, be locked away.

Consider Prescribers of Controlled Substances All practitioners who prescribe controlled substances must register with the DEA. These practitioners are authorized to prescribe controlled substances by the jurisdiction in which they are licensed. Examples of practitioners include physicians, physician assistants, nurse practitioners, dentists, veterinarians, and podiatrists. Prescribing privileges for controlled substances also depend on state laws and regulations.

Consider Prescriptions for Controlled Substances Prescriptions for a controlled substance must be written for a legitimate medical purpose. Controlled substances in Schedules III–V may only be written, faxed, or communicated verbally. In most cases, prescriptions for Schedule II controlled substances may only be delivered as handwritten prescriptions. There are a few exceptions to this rule: in an emergency, a prescriber can call in a prescription for a Schedule II controlled substance if the prescriber follows up by sending a written prescription to the pharmacy within seven days. Generally, these are for only several days' worth of medication. The other exception is for patients in hospice care, for whom prescriptions for Schedule II medications may be faxed.

Pharmacy technicians must be mindful of red flags when receiving and handling prescriptions for controlled substances. Since there is such high abuse of these medications, there is a higher risk of forged or altered prescriptions. The National Association of Boards of Pharmacy developed a video to help identify these red flags; you can view it at https://SSPharm.ParadigmEducation.com/NABP.

Consider Storage and Tracking of Controlled Substances The DEA requires controlled substances to be kept in a securely locked location in the pharmacy. In addition to the procedures dictated by federal regulations, healthcare facilities may have additional procedures to ensure the tracking of controlled substances. In some facilities, pharmacy technicians routinely count the tablets of a controlled substance prescription twice to ensure accuracy, and a pharmacist counts the tablets a third time. Each filled prescription for a controlled substance is recorded, and Schedule II drugs are recorded in a perpetual inventory logbook.

Consider the Prescription Drug Monitoring Program All states have authorized their narcotic and controlled substances agencies to use a Prescription Drug Monitoring Program (PDMP). This program is an electronic database designed to offer healthcare professionals access to a regional, multistate database of controlled substance prescription data to help make decisions about dispensing controlled substances. This information helps healthcare professionals reduce overprescribing and duplication in controlled substance prescriptions, which helps to curb controlled substance abuse.

Prescribers can review patients' prescribing histories, helping to prevent "doctor shopping," in which a patient goes to multiple doctors to get multiple prescriptions for the same medication. Pharmacy technicians can also check the PDMP when presented with a controlled substance prescription. If there are multiple prescriptions in the system for the same patient, the pharmacist can choose not to fill it.

Consider DEA Oversight of Pharmacies All pharmacies must be registered with the DEA to receive narcotics and other controlled substances from drug wholesalers. Wholesalers must also be registered with the DEA. These wholesalers, under federal law, are required to contact the DEA if they observe "unusual amounts, patterns, or frequency of drug shipments" to pharmacies. If fraudulent activity is occurring at a pharmacy, the DEA has the ability to inspect the facility. The DEA works closely with state drug and narcotic agencies that are responsible for annual physical inspections and local investigation of unsafe prescribing and dispensing of medications or forging of controlled drug prescriptions. The DEA has established an audit trail to allow the agency to track the flow of narcotics from manufacturer to warehouse to pharmacy to patient, which can be found at https://SSPharm.ParadigmEducation.com/DCD.

Many pharmacies maintain a perpetual inventory record (or tablet-by-tablet records) for complete accountability of narcotic drugs.

Because pharmacy technicians have access to controlled substance inventories, they should learn to recognize drug diversion tactics. **Diversion** describes theft of an item. Technicians who are responsible for maintaining accurate inventory records must report losses to the pharmacist in charge.

Understanding OBRA '90

The Omnibus Budget Reconciliation Act of 1990 (OBRA '90) requires states to have a Drug Utilization Review (DUR) Board, which establishes a state Medicaid preferred drug list and sets standards for pharmacist-to-patient education and counseling. This act also requires pharmacy personnel to make reasonable efforts to collect, update, and record all pertinent information in a patient's medication history.

A pharmacist must review the patient profile—known as a *DUR review*—before a prescription is filled and offer medication counseling. The offer must be documented, and the note must indicate whether the offer was accepted or refused. It is a technician's responsibility to follow established protocols in the dispensing and sale of a prescription to ensure that counseling was offered to the patient.

Understanding HIPAA

The Health Insurance Portability and Accountability Act (HIPAA) of 1996 implemented safeguards to protect patient confidentiality and protected health information, which is a patient's private medical information. The law requires that every healthcare facility—including pharmacies—have a policy on patient confidentiality that must be provided to each patient. Pharmacy technicians typically have patients sign an acknowledgement to document the receipt of this information. More information on HIPAA can be found in Module 5.

HIPAA also requires that all pharmacy personnel follow protocols for assembling and organizing patient profiles and, under penalty of law, must not reveal any information about any patient outside the pharmacy workplace. They may not discuss or transmit prescription information to anyone other than the patient, parents of children under age 18, and appropriate healthcare providers.

HIPAA is also why there are specific trash receptacles for items that include patient information, such as vial labels, monographs, and faxes. The documents in these receptacles are shredded and not placed in regular waste bins.

Pharmacies must conduct HIPAA training for personnel, appoint a privacy officer, and conduct risk analyses to comply with HIPAA.

Conduct HIPAA Training for Personnel All pharmacies must have a training program on patient data privacy for its employees, and training must be renewed annually. Training is usually written or delivered online. Such training provides technicians with examples of HIPAA violations, describes the protocols in place at the facility to protect patient information, and explains the consequences for violations.

Appoint a Privacy Officer A privacy officer ensures that proper privacy procedures are implemented, including documentation, filing, and patient requests. This individual also monitors any changes to HIPAA legislation. Much like a safety compliance or quality assurance officer, privacy officers are tasked with ensuring compliance with the most current iterations of HIPAA policies and procedures.

Conduct Risk Analyses A pharmacy manager is responsible for conducting risk analyses to identify any issues concerning patients' electronic protected health information (ePHI). These analyses must be ongoing because new technology or changes in procedures can affect privacy safeguards. The analysis reviews all existing policies, procedures, technologies, and practices used in a given setting and determines the security risk level for patient information. The manager then makes suggestions or creates action plans as necessary to ensure that ePHI is not compromised.

7.8 Federal Laws and Regulations Related to Medication Safety

Medications can have profound effects on the human body, and their use must be monitored diligently. Abuse and addiction, as well as manufacturing defects, can affect the safety of both prescription and OTC medications. When patients become addicted to a medication, their safety, as well as the safety of others affected by the abuse, becomes a critical issue.

Manufacturing defects can cause adulteration or chemical impurities during a production run for a medication. FDA regulations regarding recalls are in place to deal with them as they occur. Some of the federal laws and regulations related to medication safety include the Combat Methamphetamine Epidemic Act of 2005 and the FDA's Drug Recall Program.

Understanding the Combat Methamphetamine Epidemic Act of 2005

Sudafed and other products containing pseudoephedrine and ephedrine were once completely available as OTC medications. They are very effective for decongestant purposes and seemed relatively safe for public use, much like allergy and cold medications. However, some people started to use these medications to make methamphetamine, also known as *meth* or *speed*. Illegal drug users and dealers started to buy enormous quantities of pseudoephedrine and ephedrine from pharmacies—hundreds of dollars' worth, in some cases.

The Combat Methamphetamine Epidemic Act of 2005 reclassifies all products containing pseudoephedrine and ephedrine and restricts the amount that can be purchased at one time or in any 30-day period.

The effect of this act is that pharmacy personnel must store these products behind the counter and keep a log of all sales. Personnel must also undergo training for the handling of products containing pseudoephedrine and ephedrine. State laws and regulations for enforcing the Combat Methamphetamine Epidemic Act vary. In most cases, consumers who purchase these products must present legal identification for purchase and are allowed to purchase only a specified quantity within a certain time frame. The DEA oversees pharmacy compliance with this legislation. Pharmacy technicians should understand the laws that apply in their states and know the process for verifying identification and recording the sale into the state's system. If there is a violation of these regulations, such as a patient coming into the same store multiple times, the technician must notify the pharmacist in charge to determine the next course of action.

Understanding the FDA's Drug Recall Program

When manufacturers recall a medication, it is to remove a defective or harmful product from the market. The company may initiate the recall, or the FDA may request the recall. When it is initiated, notifications go out to all practicing pharmacies and those who may have the medication in stock.

Pharmacy technicians check computerized inventory records and pull the affected products from inventory shelves, unit-dose carts, crash carts, automated dispensing cabinets, and robots. Technicians must compare the lot number of the recalled drug with the inventory. Often recalls do not involve the entire medication in circulation but only specific lots. Typically, the technician needs to complete a form for the wholesaler that indicates the drug, strength, amount, and lot number; the products are then typically returned to the manufacturer or wholesaler for credit. In rare cases, the FDA may issue a Class I recall, which seeks to not only remove the affected lot numbers from the market but also from the patients to whom it may have been dispensed. In such cases, pharmacy technicians might assist in collecting data and reaching out to patients with further instructions.

7.9 Federal Laws and Regulations Related to Insurance Processing

Submitting insurance claims is a regular part of the work of a pharmacy technician. The pharmacy submits an electronic claim to the insurance company, which then reviews the prescriptions and judges, based on the drug coverage plan the patient has, whether a payment should be made and how much it should be. Usually, the insurance company pays the pharmacy on behalf of the patient for part of the patient's prescription cost, and the patient pays a portion as well.

Medicare is the federal government program that provides insurance for individuals older than 65, those who are under 65 and receiving disability insurance, and those under 65 with end-stage renal disease. Medicare is essentially a government insurance program, and the Medicare Modernization Act of 2003 relates specifically to pharmacy technicians.

Understanding the Medicare Modernization Act of 2003

The Medicare Modernization Act (MMA) of 2003 updated the Medicare system and initiated the option of a prescription drug insurance program called Medicare Part D. This program is suited to patients with economic hardships or patients needing high-cost medications. This legislation also launched Medicare Part C, a program that provides a comprehensive healthcare insurance option.

Practicing the Medicare Modernization Act of 2003

The MMA encourages pharmacists to provide annual in-depth reviews of the medication profiles of Medicare patients taking high-cost medications or experiencing certain chronic health conditions. The pharmacist can then look for drug interactions, adverse reactions, and ways to reduce medication costs—and get reimbursement for performing these reviews. Pharmacy technicians should be aware that Medicare Part D is a supplement to Medicare that patients pay for separately.

7.10 Professional Practice Standards

Professional practice standards, like legal guidelines, establish conduct for pharmacy personnel. For example, the National Association of Boards of Pharmacy published the "Model State Pharmacy Act." It includes standards and recommended language for state boards to use when crafting their own pharmacy legislation. The following is an example of a standard from this document regarding renewal of licenses: "Each Pharmacist, Pharmacy Intern, and Certified Pharmacy Technician shall apply for renewal of his or her license annually [or at such interval determined by the board]."

Understanding Professional Guidelines

While this standard is ideal, it is also a **guideline**, meaning it does not have to be used, unlike a state law that sets a mandatory renewal period that may differ in length. It is what may also be referred to as a **best practice**.

These types of standards are set by professional pharmacy practice organizations. The standards help to identify best practices that follow legal and ethical guidelines.

Identifying Professional Standards Organizations

Practice Tip

Knowing these organizations allows you to understand why a policy or procedure has been enacted in your pharmacy, and they can be used as resources when developing new protocols.

Many pharmacy organizations exist at both the state and national level, and their goal is to set the standard for the processes technicians use in a variety of practice settings. Some of the most well-known organizations include the following:

- National Association of Boards of Pharmacy
- American Pharmacists Association
- Institute for Safe Medication Practices
- United States Pharmacopeia (USP)
- Joint Commission
- American Society of Health-System Pharmacists (ASHP)
- Pharmacy Technician Educators Council

7.11 Ethical Standards

Ethical standards provide a moral framework for professional behavior and actions. They work in conjunction with professional practice standards to guide the behaviors of pharmacy personnel and underscore doing the right thing. Pharmacy has long been considered one of the most trustworthy professions, and highly ethical practices are what help maintain this status among patients and consumers. Ethical behaviors include obeying the federal and state laws and regulations outlined above.

Adhering to an Ethical Code of Conduct

Ethical codes of behavior in pharmacy are based on trust. Patients put their trust in the knowledge, competency, honesty, and integrity of pharmacy personnel to serve their unique healthcare needs and to ensure the safety of their health and well-being. For these reasons, pharmacy personnel must be held to high standards of professional behavior. Laws and regulations governing pharmacy practice dictate the legal course of action but do not always dictate the proper route to take in a course of action. Ethics play a role in guiding the decision-making and actions of pharmacy personnel.

A code of ethics regarding professional behavior is often written as a formal document and supported by professional organizations. The statements that make up the code provide language to aid in the decision-making process when an ethical issue presents itself in pharmacy practice. They are sets of rules that can be used as a deciding factor if the answer to a problem or issue is not clear. The American Association of Pharmacy Technicians (AAPT), the American Society of Health-System Pharmacists (ASHP), and the Pharmacy Technician Certification Board (PTCB) have published a code of ethics for pharmacy personnel.

> "A code of ethics regarding professional behavior is often written as a formal document and supported by professional organizations."

While the language may vary, these codes of conduct follow the same overarching principles and guidelines. Many of the codes are meant to help technicians follow the laws listed earlier in this chapter as well as guide professional conduct to ensure the best outcomes for patient care. If these codes are followed, you will perform your duties and responsibilities in the most ethical and professional manner possible. Below are links to these codes of conduct.

- AAPT Codes of Conduct: https://SSPharm.ParadigmEducation.com/AAPTConduct
- ASHP Codes of Conduct: https://SSPharm.ParadigmEducation.com/ASHPConduct
- PTCB Codes of Conduct: https://SSPharm.ParadigmEducation.com/PTCBConduct

Think It Through: Codes of Conduct

Think about your current approach and mind-set when making decisions. Do you have a personal code of conduct that influences what decisions you make and how you behave? If you do, how well does it align with your career as a pharmacy technician?

Self-Reflection: Do You Behave Ethically?

For each of the statements, answer "always," "sometimes," or "rarely/never" to rate your ethical decision-making skills. Respond to statements as honestly as possible.

When considering my own ethical decision-making skills, I…	Always	Sometimes	Rarely/Never
take time to consider situations before making a decision.			
gather information from multiple sources.			
consider the accuracy of various sources.			
know my employer's policies and procedures.			
follow my employer's policies and procedures.			
consider all parties involved in the decision.			
identify the positive consequences of potential decisions.			
identify the negative consequences of potential decisions.			
confidently choose a course of action.			
follow up on the outcomes of a decision.			
make necessary changes after reviewing a decision.			
Subtotal per column	_____ x5	_____ x3	_____ x1

Tally Your Score: Always = 5 points; Sometimes = 3 points; Rarely/Never = 1 point

Total Score: _____

34 to 55 points: This score indicates that you have a strong ethical framework for decision-making.

12 to 33 points: This score indicates that your ethical framework is satisfactory but could be improved.

Below 12 points: This score indicates that your ethical framework is not strong; you should identify areas that need work.

Building an Ethical Framework

There will be many times in your career when you will be faced with several options to choose from. There may not be a clear right or wrong answer in these cases—merely the best or most ethical option. Selecting the best option requires the ability to make distinctions between these competing options. There are seven steps to aid in making ethical choices: stop and think, determine the facts, follow facility regulations, consider all affected individuals, weigh the consequences, make the decision, and review the results of your decision.

As we use these steps, consider the following hypothetical ethical scenario:

A patient comes to the counter very agitated and needs to know if a drug he is currently taking will interact with an OTC medication he wants to purchase. The patient is late for a job interview, and the pharmacist has stepped out to use the restroom. You happen to know the answer to the question, and the pharmacist has told you to relay the information in the past to another patient. Do you tell the patient the information you remember from the last time?

Stop and Think This advice may seem obvious, but slowing down and taking time to stop and think through your options will prevent you from making snap or rash decisions. There is nothing wrong with saying, "I need time to think about this situation."

In the example, asking the patient to wait while you go and see if the pharmacist is available (even though you know she is not) can buy you time to consider your options.

Determine the Facts You should have all relevant and important information to support an intelligent decision. To determine whether you have all the facts, make a list of what is known and unknown to you. If needed, seek additional information and verify (or dismiss) assumptions and other uncertain information. Additionally, it is important to consider the reliability and credibility of the people providing this information.

Knowing what the patient is purchasing and what it is used for, you can determine if the need is critical enough to relay what you already know without pharmacist direction or if the patient can wait or come back after his interview.

Follow Facility Regulations Pharmacy personnel must follow their facility's policy and procedures manual to ensure the ethical operation of the pharmacy. If an option does not align with the policies and procedures, it should be discarded.

While you can relay information to a patient upon pharmacist direction, doing so unaided is considered counseling and is against facility and legal regulations.

Consider All Affected Individuals When deciding, you must think about *all* the individuals who will potentially be affected by the decision. Often there are more people that can be affected than initially considered.

In the scenario, you would be affected by a potential reprimand or termination, but the patient could also be affected. In this case, he could either miss his job interview while having to wait or be given incorrect information that could lead to a medication error.

Weigh the Consequences Often there will be outcomes both positive and negative in deciding a course of action. Filter your choices to determine if any of your options will violate any core ethical values, and then eliminate the unethical options.

If you decide to help the patient, you may make his day easier and perform what could be perceived as good customer service, which could result in a repeat customer. However, you could also be terminated or cause a serious medication error from choosing to counsel him. If you choose not to assist him and ask him to wait or come back, you might lose him as a customer but would not face the other consequences.

Make the Decision Ultimately, you must decide. If you are still struggling to see a clear choice, try talking with others who may be involved or affected to get their opinions. Seek the advice of individuals you respect and trust, including people you know who have a strong moral compass. Ask yourself, "If everyone found out about my decision, would I be proud and comfortable with it?"

Review the Results of Your Decision Ethical decision-makers monitor the effects of their choices and learn from their mistakes. If your decision is not producing the intended results or is causing undesirable results, reassess the situation and make a new decision.

7.12 Module Summary

Laws are what guide our conduct and ensure safety and prosperity. This statement holds true for the practice of pharmacy as well. To effectively carry out our duties, we must understand the laws at both the state and federal levels that regulate our scope of practice. As pharmacy technicians assume more advanced responsibilities, they will have more legal liability. Pharmacy personnel must adhere to all federal and state laws and regulations or risk legal repercussions. Violations in laws may result in damages, fines, probation, loss of licensure, or—in extreme cases—incarceration. It is also necessary to follow an ethical framework in the interpretation and execution of these laws and regulations. By following a code of conduct, pharmacy technicians can conduct themselves with the highest level of professionalism.

 The online course includes additional review and assessment resources.

Externship Preparation & Practice

LEARNING OBJECTIVES

1   Define the terms *experiential learning* and preceptor. (Introduction)

2   Recognize the benefits that an externship provides to students and to practice sites (Section 8.1).

3   Understand the general externship requirements, including the submission of personal identification and educational documentation. (Section 8.2)

4   Know the experiential hour requirements and program levels for schools accredited by ASHP/ACPE. (Section 8.2)

5   Learn the program-specific externship requirements, including knowledge of learning objectives, responsibilities of externs, related externship assignments, required hours, state pharmacy laws and regulations, and provisions for transportation and childcare. (Section 8.3)

6   Understand pre-externship health screening requirements, including a physical exam, an immunization update, and a urine drug test. (Section 8.4)

7   Recognize the components of a criminal background check, a mandatory procedure for externship participation. (Section 8.4)

8   Understand your externship assignment, including the rotation requirements, preceptor/extern professional relationship, work schedule, and evaluation and grading parameters. (Section 8.5)

9   Prepare for an initial meeting with your preceptor and a facility orientation. (Section 8.5)

10 Know the professional and technical competencies expected of an extern. (Section 8.6)

To view the *ASHP/ACPE Accreditation Standards* addressed in this chapter, refer to Appendix A.

As a pharmacy technician student, you must fulfill the education and training requirements established by your state's board of pharmacy. In addition, if your academic program adheres to the standards of the American Society of Health-System Pharmacists (ASHP) and the Accreditation Council for Pharmacy Education (ACPE), you must also complete an experiential learning experience in an actual pharmacy setting. **Experiential learning** is a process through which you will further develop the knowledge and skills of a pharmacy technician while engaged in a professional work environment. Consequently, experiential learning is considered "learning by doing" and is referred to by many names: *externship*, *internship*, *apprenticeship*, *practice experience*, or *practicum*. For pharmacy technician programs, the most commonly used term is *externship*.

A pharmacy externship site has a seasoned pharmacy professional, such as a pharmacist or another pharmacy technician, who serves as a **preceptor**. This individual is responsible for your training while participating in an externship and serves as the primary contact between the school and the practice site. As part of those responsibilities, a preceptor coordinates your schedule, signs your time sheets, conducts your midterm and final evaluations, and oversees your training.

This module walks you through several stages of the externship process. Some of the topics include general and program-specific externship requirements, registration paperwork, prerequisite health screening and background checks, preceptor assignment and initial meeting, facility orientation, and expected technical and professional competencies of an extern.

8.1 Benefits of an Externship

As mentioned earlier, an externship provides you with the opportunity to step into the role of a pharmacy technician in a variety of settings. Under the guidance of a preceptor, you will apply the knowledge, skills, and abilities you learned in your academic program to your technician responsibilities in a pharmacy setting. This authentic experience is beneficial to your professional development. However, you may be surprised to learn that your externship may also be beneficial to the practice site itself.

Recognizing Student Benefits

The student benefits of an externship are considerable. The experience allows you to assess your current knowledge and skills, gain real-world pharmacy experience, undergo pharmacy software training, learn from the guidance of a professional mentor, and profit from networking opportunities.

Assesses Your Current Knowledge and Skills Participating in an externship is a means to gauge your ability to apply your academic knowledge. The experience also allows you to practice your soft skills and professionalism while performing daily tasks and interacting with patients. Consequently, your externship helps you to assess the proficiencies and deficiencies of your knowledge, skills, and abilities. This assessment, in turn, helps you to improve those areas of deficiency as you prepare for the national certification exam and your entrance into the job market.

Provides Real-World Pharmacy Practice An externship offers you an authentic pharmacy practice experience. This experience is different from the simulated practice environment that was part of your academic instruction. One difference is that you will gain experience with site-specific technologies and processes that may not be covered in your academic coursework. Another distinction is that real-world practice has real-life consequences for patients. For that reason, you must seek frequent guidance and feedback from your preceptor and pharmacy colleagues as you perform your daily responsibilities.

Another benefit of an authentic pharmacy practice experience is that the training provides you with a level of comfort prior to securing an entry-level position. You gain experience in several areas: daily operations of a pharmacy, roles of pharmacy staff members, interprofessional skills, customer service relations, time management, efficiency, problem-solving scenarios, conflict management, and proficiency in dispensing medications.

Supplies Pharmacy Software Training An externship provides you with training in the use of pharmacy software programs. These programs support different pharmacy operations, depending on the setting. Such operations include entering prescription data, printing prescription medication labels, using a retail point-of-sale system, conducting inventory, and tracking medications. These programs also serve as databases of patients, prescribers, medications, and insurance companies. Examples of commonly used pharmacy software programs include the following:

- Pyxis
- Siemens Pharmacy
- PioneerRx
- NRx (QS/1)
- Rx30
- Omnicell

Be aware that the programs listed above reflect a portion of available pharmacy software. In addition, many pharmacies have their own proprietary software programs that they use in their daily operations. Consequently, the pharmacy software program that you learn during your externship may or may not be the program used at the pharmacy where you secure your entry-level position. The good news is that all pharmacy software programs are designed to essentially perform the same functions. Therefore, if you learn one system, it becomes much easier to learn another one.

Provides a Professional Mentor As mentioned earlier, your externship program is under the tutelage of a preceptor. This experienced individual serves as a **professional mentor** and externship supervisor who provides guidance, advice, and support during your externship. Once your externship is completed, your preceptor will be an invaluable resource for career opportunities and provide a reference for your career portfolio. For that reason, make every effort to establish a strong, positive, professional relationship with your mentor. (See the section titled "Meeting Your Preceptor" for information on this professional relationship.)

Other pharmacy employees you work with during your externship will also provide you with guidance during your training. Make every effort to establish good relationships with your colleagues and seek their guidance as needed.

> ### Think It Through: Building Your Pharmacy Relationships
> Consider how you interact with individuals in positions of authority: supervisors, instructors, coaches, etc. What aspects of these interactions can you bring to your relationship with a preceptor? How can you demonstrate initiative to a preceptor and other pharmacy employees during an externship?

Offers Networking Opportunities An externship is an opportunity for you to demonstrate your knowledge, skills, and professional demeanor to a potential employer. For that reason, consider your externship as a "working interview" for a potential position after you graduate. Your demonstrated job competencies and interactions with your colleagues and patients provide a pharmacy manager with insight into how well suited you are for employment at that facility.

Even if that pharmacy does not have an opening when you begin your job search, the relationships that you establish with the healthcare staff (e.g., preceptor, pharmacy colleagues, providers, nurses) form a professional network that may assist you in launching your career. Be sure to ask individuals whom you have closely worked with during your externship for contact information and references before completing your externship.

Recognizing Practice Site Benefits

The practice site itself benefits from participating in pharmacy technician externships in conjunction with academic programs. These benefits include an increase in staffing, an investment in the pharmacy profession, and an enhanced public image.

Provides Additional Staff While participating in your externship, you are considered a contributing staff member. You provide an extra pair of hands to assist pharmacy personnel in meeting the healthcare needs of customers and patients. Although initially your training may have a minimal positive impact on pharmacy procedures, you will, with time, learn the facility's operations and become comfortable and competent in your responsibilities. You will fall into the rhythm of the daily tasks and work collaboratively with your preceptor and your colleagues to provide customer and patient healthcare services.

WORKPLACE WISDOM

Leveling Up

Be aware that the initial phase of your training may slow down pharmacy operations. Your training may also test the patience of some colleagues, who may be used to working with personnel who know the ins and outs of that facility's processes. However, with time, that phase will transition to a more collaborative practice environment. As you become versed in the processes and procedures, your presence will speed up operations. Remember to always give your maximum effort while working to compensate for any decrease in efficiency in the early stages of your training.

Invests in the Future of the Pharmacy Profession A pharmacy's externship program keeps the pharmacy profession moving forward. Pharmacy technician students who have a positive externship experience are inclined to continue in the profession and secure its future success. Employers that train students, even if they are unable to employ them at their facility, help improve the quality of every pharmacy technician who comes through their facility. This training helps to raise the level of competency for technicians throughout the industry.

Enhances Public Image An externship practice site is an investment in the local community. The relationship between the school and the pharmacy promotes the pharmacy's views on the importance of education. In addition, the facility's willingness to hire community members at the completion of an externship emphasizes this relationship.

8.2 General Externship Requirements

General externship requirements vary among states, schools, employers, and practice sites. For that reason, check with your externship coordinator for the externship requirements associated with your program. Often, these requirements are addressed in an orientation just before your externship begins. Basic requirements include the submission of proper identification (ID) and academic documentation. In addition, if your school is accredited by ASHP/ACPE, you must fulfill the externship requirements set by those organizations.

Completing Basic Requirements

Submitting the required documentation within the allotted time frame designated by your school is critical. This documentation typically includes a proper means of personal ID, your educational documents, and—in some states—evidence of your state registration or licensure. This evidence may be a technician-in-training license or registration. Again, verify the necessary paperwork with your externship coordinator due to variance among states and academic institutions.

Present Personal ID You are required to submit proof of personal ID before beginning a pharmacy technician externship. The following items may be submitted: a driver's license, a photo ID card (such as a school ID card), or a Social Security card. Some schools require a current photo ID for students participating in an externship.

Submit Educational Documents To participate in a pharmacy technician externship, you must meet your state requirements for eligibility. These requirements may vary, but typically you must be enrolled in a high school program, have attained a high school diploma, or have passed a general educational development (GED) test. You must also be actively enrolled in a pharmacy technician program, have taken your program's required prerequisite courses, and have earned the stated grade minimums (typically a C or higher) in these courses.

Submit State Registration and Certification Documents Before participating in an externship, some states require that you are registered as a pharmacy technician trainee and licensed with the state, with no suspension, limitation, revocation, or denial of your registration or licensure. In some states, this license may be called a *technician-in-training license*, which is similar to a learner's permit for driving. It allows you to perform technician duties while learning under the supervision of others. Once you have fulfilled your course of study, this technician-in-training license converts to a full pharmacy technician license. The acquisition of this registration or license is typically handled by the externship coordinator in your program of study.

Fulfilling ASHP/ACPE Standards

All pharmacy technician programs that have earned accreditation by the **American Society of Health-System Pharmacists (ASHP)** and the **Accreditation Council for Pharmacy Education (ACPE)** must adhere to the organizations' standards for the fulfillment of a pharmacy technician externship. The *ASHP/ACPE Accreditation Standards* are developed to do the following:

- protect the public by ensuring the availability of a competent workforce
- describe pharmacy technician education and training program development at the entry level and the advanced level
- provide criteria for the evaluation of new and established education and training programs
- promote continuous improvement of established educational and training programs

These standards state that an externship must be an authentic, hands-on experience under the supervision of a preceptor. An externship *cannot* be a job-shadowing or simulated experience. As such, you are given the opportunity to practice most of the activities that pharmacy technicians perform daily in a given setting. One of the few areas you may not be allowed to practice would be the handling of money during dispensing transactions. Because you are considered a pharmacy team member during your externship, you must abide by the policies and procedures of the practice site.

Understand ASHP/ACPE Program Levels The current *ASHP/ACPE Accreditation Standards* include two levels of pharmacy education and training: entry level and advanced level. These levels can be offered sequentially or concurrently. The term *sequentially* means that you must complete the entry-level coursework before you are eligible to pursue the advanced-level coursework. The other option that schools have is to offer both levels simultaneously as part of an all-inclusive program. These levels reflect the expected competencies needed in entry-level and advanced-level roles in a variety of pharmacy settings (e.g., community, institutional, home care, long-term care).

The entry-level and advanced-level programs share a similar framework. Both programs have three educational components: didactic, simulated, and experiential. The **didactic educational component** is the instruction that provides a foundation for the simulated and experiential components. It is the knowledge learned in an academic setting. The **simulated educational component** refers to hands-on practice in a simulated pharmacy environment, such as a school lab, that has no real-world consequences. The **experiential educational component** is an externship experience in a real-world pharmacy setting.

Entry-Level Program If you are enrolled in an entry-level program, you need to obtain 400 health-related curriculum hours over a period of eight weeks, of which 300 hours are specified by educational modality:

- didactic: 120 hours
- simulated: 50 hours
- experiential: 130 hours

The remaining 100 hours may be allocated to any of these three modalities, as specified by your academic program. When you have finished your entry-level program, you are issued a certificate of completion or a diploma.

Advanced-Level Program If you are enrolled in an advanced-level program, you must obtain an additional 200 health-related curriculum hours over a period of at least seven weeks, of which 160 hours are specified by educational modality:

- didactic: 40 hours
- simulated: 50 hours
- experiential: 70 hours

The remaining 40 hours may be allocated to any of these three modalities, as specified by your academic program. When you have finished your advanced-level program, you are issued a certificate of completion or a diploma.

8.3 Program-Specific Externship Requirements

Your program director, adviser, or externship coordinator typically meets with you to discuss program-specific externship requirements. This discussion may address the learning objectives of an externship and the student responsibilities while working at the pharmacy site.

Understanding the Learning Objectives of an Externship

Before beginning an externship, you should be familiar with the learning objectives that your school has established for this experience. **Learning objectives** are statements that define what is meant to be learned in a given course of study. These learning objectives are based on the skill sets that pharmacy technicians must demonstrate in a workplace. These objectives will appear in your course syllabus as well as in your midterm and final evaluations completed by your preceptor. Review these learning objectives before starting your externship to ensure that you understand the expectations of this experiential learning experience. Also, periodically review the skill sets during your externship to gauge your level of competency and to target areas for growth or improvement before starting your career search.

Ticking All the Right Boxes

To give you an overview of the goals of a pharmacy technician externship program, refer to the following set of learning objectives from Austin Community College in Texas. Be aware that learning objectives vary among academic institutions and states.

❑ assist the pharmacist in collecting, organizing, and evaluating information for direct patient care, medication use review, and departmental management

❑ receive and screen prescriptions/medication orders for completeness and authenticity

❑ prepare medications for distribution

❑ verify the measurements, preparation, and/or packaging of medications produced by other pharmacy technicians

❑ distribute medications

❑ assist the pharmacist in the administration of immunizations

❑ assist the pharmacist in the identification of patients who desire/require counseling

❑ initiate, verify, assist in the adjudication of, and collect payment and/or initiate billing for pharmacy services and goods

❑ purchase pharmaceuticals, devices, and supplies

❑ control the inventory of medications, equipment, and devices according to an established plan

❑ assist the pharmacist in monitoring the practice site for compliance with federal, state, and local laws, regulations, and professional standards

❑ maintain pharmacy equipment and facilities

❑ assist the pharmacist in preparing, storing, and distributing investigational medication products

❑ assist the pharmacist in monitoring medication therapy

❑ participate in the pharmacy department's process for preventing medication misadventures

❑ take personal responsibility for assisting the pharmacist in improving direct patient care

❑ demonstrate ethical conduct

❑ maintain a professional image

❑ resolve conflicts through negotiation

❑ understand the principles for managing change

❑ appreciate the need to adapt direct patient care to meet the needs of diversity

❑ appreciate the benefits of involvement in local, state, and national pharmacy organizations

❑ appreciate the value of obtaining pharmacy technician certification

❑ understand the importance of staying current with changes in pharmacy practice

❑ communicate clearly when speaking or writing

❑ maximize work efficiency through the use of technology

❑ efficiently solve problems in one's work

❑ display a caring attitude toward patients

❑ maintain confidentiality of patient and proprietary business information

❑ understand direct patient care delivery systems in multiple practice settings

❑ efficiently manage one's work, whether performed alone or as part of a team

❑ function effectively as a healthcare team member

❑ balance obligations to one's self, relationships, and work in a way that minimizes stress

❑ understand the use and side effects of prescription medications, nonprescription medications, and alternative therapies (e.g., herbal products, dietary supplements, homeopathy, lifestyle modification) used to treat common disease states

❑ assist the pharmacist in assuring the quality of all pharmaceutical services

Adapted and used with permission from Austin Community College, Austin, Texas

Understanding the Responsibilities of Externs

Your coordinator will discuss with you the related items that must be completed during your externship. These items may include progress reports, interviews, time sheets, evaluations, and competencies. You are responsible for the completion and timely submission of these items. In addition, you are accountable for fulfilling the required number of externship hours for the program, knowing your state's pharmacy laws and regulations, observing patient privacy standards, and arranging transportation and childcare (if applicable) during this practice experience.

Learn the Related Externship Assignments Your program may require you to complete related assignments while participating in your externship. These assignments factor into your final grade for that term and may include any or all of the following activities:

- weekly progress reports
- weekly time sheets
- daily journal entries
- competency checklists
- quizzes and final exam
- self-evaluation survey of your experience
- summary written report of your experience
- updated résumé, which includes your externship experience
- mock pre-employment interview

Make sure that you are aware of any assigned activities, including their guidelines, due dates, and percentage of your final grade.

Complete the Required Hours The number of externship hours that must be completed are determined by your school and, possibly, your state board of pharmacy. As mentioned earlier, institutions accredited by ASHP/ACPE must adhere to the minimum number of experiential hours required by these organizations: 130 hours for entry-level programs and 70 hours for advanced-level programs. However, many of these accredited schools require additional experiential hours than the ASHP/ACPE standards state.

Your school also determines the number of weeks per term and the minimum number of hours per week for pharmacy technician externships. To document your experiential hours, you will complete daily or weekly time sheets that will be signed by your preceptor and reviewed by your externship coordinator. (For more information on time sheets, refer to the section titled "Meeting Your Preceptor.")

Know Your State's Pharmacy Laws and Regulations As a pharmacy extern, you are required to follow your state board of pharmacy's laws and regulations during your externship. For example, in some states, you must maintain an active registration as a pharmacy technician or technician-in-training during your experiential rotation(s). Other states have different requirements for pharmacy externs. For that reason, be sure to investigate what is needed for registration or licensure before your practice experience.

No matter where you reside, you must adhere to the scope of practice set forth by your state's board of pharmacy. Scope of practice determines what responsibilities pharmacy technicians may assume. These responsibilities vary among states; for example, pharmacy technicians in Idaho are allowed to administer immunizations. For that reason, familiarize yourself with state laws that dictate what you can and cannot do in a pharmacy setting. Your preceptor will also provide guidance regarding scope of practice during your externship. (For more information on scope of practice, see Module 7.)

> "No matter where you reside, you must adhere to the scope of practice set forth by your state's board of pharmacy."

Observe Patient and Pharmacy Confidentiality Standards As a pharmacy extern, you are required to uphold the patient confidentiality standards dictated by the Health Insurance Portability and Accountability Act (HIPAA) of 1996. These standards prohibit the acquisition, access, use, or disclosure of patient health information and patient records by any means: electronic, written, or verbal communication. This legislation also does not allow you, as an extern, to access your own medical records under any circumstance.

You must also adhere to these pharmacy confidentiality standards during your externship. While all pharmacies in the country must follow the law regarding HIPAA, the procedures in which they do so may vary. In some facilities, pharmacy personnel discard documents containing patient information in dedicated, color-coded shred bins. Personnel in other pharmacies may use a separate garbage bin devoted to the disposal of patient documents. Patient acknowledgment of privacy laws may differ among pharmacies as well. In some facilities, pharmacy personnel ask patients to provide an electronic signature as verification of their understanding of HIPAA standards. Personnel in other pharmacies may ask patients to sign a paper logbook. Be sure that you know the policies of your practice site regarding the disposal of patient information and the patient acknowledgment of HIPAA standards.

Find Transportation You are responsible for your transportation to and from the externship practice site(s). If you do not have access to a vehicle, you may

Work Wise

You may be required to complete an online HIPAA training course before the start of your externship, or you may receive your training during the didactic component of your academic program. Check with your school to determine what type of HIPAA training is necessary.

want to research public transportation options once you receive your externship assignment. Other options include using a ride-hail service, such as Uber or Lyft, or posting your interest in ride-sharing at your school or on a social media site. Be sure to factor transportation costs into your budget for the academic term.

Secure Childcare If you need childcare, explore your options well before the start of your pharmacy externship. Having a schedule for your childcare coverage is important information to relay to your externship coordinator and to your preceptor at your initial meeting. Like your transportation costs, be sure to factor in your childcare expenditures when creating your budget for the academic term.

> ### Think It Through: Assessing Your Backup Plans
> Proper planning before the start of your externship allows you to have a successful practice experience and to make a favorable impression on a potential future employer. Consider your current schedule, responsibilities, and potential challenges that may interfere with your externship. Have you made backup plans to manage any situations or difficulties that may arise? What specific backup plans would help you navigate these possible challenges?

8.4 Pre-externship Screening

As an extern, you are not an employee of a pharmacy, but you are expected to behave as if you were. You must adhere to the facility's policies and procedures during your practice experience. For that reason, you must typically undergo a pre-externship health screening and a criminal background check before the start of your externship.

Submitting to a Health Screening

A **health screening** is required for healthcare personnel due to their preparation of medications and their contact with customers or patients. The typical components of this health screening are a physical exam, an immunization update, and a drug-screening test. Documented evidence of the results of this health screening, known as a *health screening attestation form*, must be submitted to your practice site before the start of your externship.

Your externship coordinator typically handles the submission of these forms to your practice site, but you may be responsible for their submission. If you are responsible, be sure to adhere to the established deadline of the practice site for this information.

Undergo a Physical Exam To ensure that you have the physical stamina to meet the demands of a fast-paced pharmacy environment, including long periods of standing on your feet, you will undergo a physical exam. This basic exam typically entails assessing your blood pressure, heart rate, height and weight, balance while standing, mobility, and ability to lift a minimum weight, such as 15 lbs.

Receive Required Immunizations Before the start of your externship, you must submit an up-to-date **immunization record** as proof that you have received the vaccines and tests required by your school or practice site. Because you will be in close contact with many customers and patients during your practice experience, it is important that you do not contribute to the spread of a viral or bacterial infection. The required vaccines and tests may vary among practice sites. For example, a two-step skin test or QuantiFERON-TB Gold blood screening for tuberculosis is mandatory for personnel working in a hospital setting. A current flu shot may also be required by certain pharmacy settings during flu season. Immunizations and tests that are commonly required for pharmacy personnel include the following:

- tuberculosis (purified protein derivative [PPD]—a nonreactive, two-step skin test within 90 days of the start of the externship that must not expire during the externship)
- measles, mumps, and rubella (MMR)
- chicken pox (varicella)
- flu (influenza)
- hepatitis B (series of three injections)
- tetanus, diphtheria, and pertussis (Td/Tdap)

You can receive these immunizations and tests at a physician's office, clinic, pharmacy, health center, or travel clinic. Remember that some immunizations, such as hepatitis B or the MMR booster, require a series of injections to provide immunity. For that reason, be sure to check your immunization record well ahead of the start of your externship.

If you do not have access to your immunization record, there are several ways to obtain it, depending on the state where the immunizations were administered. You can search online databases or communicate with the health department of the state where you received the immunizations to request these documents.

Take a Drug-Screening Test As part of your health screening, you are required to undergo a **drug-screening test**. This test identifies if there are illicit drugs or substances in your system. As such, this test is critical for

Practice Tip

To find a facility to obtain the required immunizations for your externship, visit the following website and enter your zip code in the Vaccine Finder: https://SSPharm .Paradigm Education .com/Immune.

pharmacy personnel due to their access to controlled substances. The fee for this test may be covered as part of your tuition, so check with your externship coordinator. If the fee is not part of your tuition, you are responsible for paying it.

Typically, the drug-screening test that is required for a pharmacy technician externship is a urine drug test. This test analyzes a urine specimen for specific drugs and chemicals, including the following:

- amphetamines
- barbiturates
- benzodiazepines
- cocaine
- marijuana
- methadone
- methamphetamines
- opioids
- phencyclidine (PCP)
- synthetic urine

The presence of any of these substances in your urine specimen, except a medication that has a valid prescription, may prevent you from participating in an externship. Consequently, the time and money that you have invested in your academic program would be wasted and have no tangible outcome.

WORKPLACE WISDOM

Taking a Urine Drug Test

You will follow a specific protocol to take a urine drug test. This protocol ensures that you are not submitting a fraudulent urine specimen for analysis. After receiving a urine specimen cup and moist cloth from the supervising technician administering the test, you will empty your pockets and place your belongings in a locker. Then you will enter the bathroom, cleanse your genitals with the moist cloth, and void a minimum of 45 mL of urine into the specimen cup. When you have finished voiding, you will place a lid on the cup. Then, without flushing the toilet, you will exit the bathroom and hand your cup to the technician. The technician will then measure the temperature of your urine to ensure that it is within the expected range for a recently voided specimen. Finally, the technician will seal and package the urine specimen in your presence and send the specimen to the laboratory.

You will also be required to take some type of drug-screening test before you begin an entry-level pharmacy position. Depending on the hiring facility, you may need to submit a urine specimen or a hair sample. Once you begin your employment, you will undergo regular or random drug-screening tests, depending on the facility's policies.

Career Readiness & Externships: Soft Skills for Pharmacy Technicians

Drug Screening and Legalized Marijuana

Your school or program of study will have a policy regarding the drug-screening process and what constitutes a failed test. Synthetic urine, controlled substances without a valid prescription, or illegal substances are all things that could constitute a failed test and prevent you from starting your externship.

Marijuana has now been legalized in many states for both recreational and medicinal use. However, marijuana is still categorized by the federal government as a Schedule I controlled substance. This dilemma is a gray area in the drug-screening process for states where marijuana use is legal. In most states where marijuana has been legalized, a positive test for marijuana can be ignored. However, this decision rests with the institution. It is entirely the school's right to expect students to not use marijuana while enrolled in their program of study. Furthermore, it is the legal right of employers to choose whether they want to employ someone who uses marijuana, despite its legality.

Check your institution's policy regarding a drug-screening test. In addition, talk with your instructor, program chair, or externship coordinator about how a drug-screening test is handled if you live in a state where marijuana is legal.

Submitting to a Criminal Background Check

As part of your prescreening employment, you are required to undergo a **criminal background check**. This procedure applies to all pharmacy employees because of their access to medications—in particular, controlled substances. A criminal background check is often performed as part of the enrollment process with a program of study or before the start of an externship. Check with your program adviser or externship coordinator to determine what actions you must take to fulfill this background check.

A background check differs among states but may include these steps:

- investigation of a criminal record (both felonies and misdemeanors)
- confirmation of an extern's educational credentials
- verification of an extern's licensure and registration
- confirmation of an extern's employment history
- investigation of an extern's credit history
- investigation of an appearance on a sex offender registry
- verification of fingerprints

Disqualifying factors for a pharmacy technician externship include a felony conviction; a suspension, denial, revocation, or limitation on your registration or licensure; or a history of drug-related offenses, including misdemeanors. In some states, such as Nevada, noncompliance with court-ordered child support can prevent a technician-in-training registration and, therefore, can prohibit an individual from completing an externship.

Self-Reflection:
Are You Ready to Begin Your Externship?

Read each statement. If you feel confident that you can say "yes" to that statement, place a check mark in the first column. For any unchecked statement, consider what steps you can take to gain self-awareness in that area.

✔	Statement
	I know the name of the externship coordinator of my pharmacy technician program.
	I know the pharmacy settings that are available for my externship.
	I have researched potential externship sites to learn more about them.
	I am familiar with the roles of pharmacy technicians in various settings.
	I understand the program-specific externship requirements of my state and school.
	I understand the need for a health screening and criminal background check before my externship.
	I feel that my knowledge and skills have prepared me for my externship responsibilities.
	I have secured reliable transportation to get to and from my practice site.
	I have arranged my schedule to ensure my availability for my externship.
	I have made backup plans for any potential challenges to the completion of my externship.
	I understand the importance of my professional conduct while participating in an externship.
	I understand the state laws and regulations that dictate the scope of practice for pharmacy technicians.

8.5 Externship Assignment

Often, a school's pharmacy technician program has several long-standing partnerships with local pharmacies that host externs for their rotations. For that reason, your externship coordinator typically arranges your externship with one of these pharmacies and then meets with you to relay the assigned practice site. When determining your placement, the coordinator considers several factors:

- your academic performance
- your punctuality and attendance
- your behavioral, social, communication, and observational skills
- your lab skills (e.g., prescription entry, pill counting, sterile compounding)

Remember that you are representing the school as well as yourself when you participate in an externship. Therefore, you must exhibit professional behaviors while working at the practice site. If your preceptor reports that you have work-related issues despite corrective feedback, you risk a possible termination from your externship. Termination from an externship site is equivalent to failing a course in your program of study. Your poor performance or unprofessional behavior also jeopardizes the school's partnership with the practice site, which may affect the externship options for future students.

WORKPLACE WISDOM

Where Will I Complete My Externship?

The externship coordinator of your pharmacy technician program may post a few practice sites on the school's website and allow you to rank available sites in terms of preference. A program that offers this privilege is not required to grant your request, just as it is not required to grant your request for a specific instructor in your academic program.

Other pharmacy technician programs may have you secure your own externship practice site. Most often, your externship coordinator or program director will discuss viable options with you based on your location, availability, and preferences and work with you to try to place you at the most optimal setting.

Learning Your Rotation Requirements

Depending on your school's program, you may be required to rotate through two different pharmacy settings, which may include a community pharmacy, institutional pharmacy, long-term care pharmacy, or mail-order pharmacy. These rotations provide you with an opportunity to use skill sets that may be specific to a certain setting. For example, participating in a community pharmacy externship hones your customer service skills. However, an institutional pharmacy externship gives you more experience with automation and sterile compounding. Your externship coordinator will let you know of the site rotation requirements for your institution.

Researching Your Practice Site

Whether you have the option of choosing your practice site or being assigned one, you should research the site before beginning your externship. Check out basic information about the facility on its website: its location, hours of operation, number of employees, and services. You may also want to review the facility's profile on various social networking sites. Becoming familiar with the pharmacy before beginning your externship provides you with a basic level of comfort regarding the pharmacy's staff and customer or patient services.

Meeting Your Preceptor

Your externship coordinator will relay the name of your preceptor at your assigned practice site. You or your coordinator will contact your preceptor to set up either the first day to start your externship or an initial meeting with your preceptor. At that meeting, your preceptor will discuss the preceptor/extern professional relationship, create a mutually agreed-upon work schedule, review evaluation and grading parameters, and conduct a facility orientation.

Discuss the Preceptor/Extern Professional Relationship As mentioned earlier in this module, your preceptor serves as a supervisor and mentor during your externship. As such, your preceptor will offer guidance to help you learn pharmacy operations and navigate professional relationships. For that reason, it is important to establish a good working relationship from the start.

At your initial meeting with your preceptor, be sure to create a good first impression by arriving on time for the meeting, exhibiting professionalism in your communications and behaviors, and demonstrating your willingness to learn more about the technician position in a pharmacy. Your preceptor, in turn, will discuss the role of a preceptor in your professional development and the expectations of the position. These expectations include your demonstration of professional and technical competencies. (For specific information on these competencies, refer to the section titled "Externship Practice.")

You can foster a good professional relationship by exhibiting the following behaviors:

- demonstrating your understanding of all federal and state laws and regulations in your daily responsibilities
- following the policies and procedures of your practice site
- being an active participant and a good listener during your experiential learning experience
- demonstrating respect for your preceptor and other healthcare colleagues while performing your daily tasks
- checking with your preceptor when making professional decisions
- asking questions of your preceptor when you need clarification on a specific task
- seeking guidance from your preceptor, as necessary, to navigate a conflict or disagreement
- using common sense when performing your work responsibilities
- learning from your preceptor's constructive criticism
- demonstrating accountability for your actions

Career Readiness & Externships: Soft Skills for Pharmacy Technicians

Create a Work Schedule You and your preceptor will create a work schedule that accommodates your other commitments (e.g., full-time job, classes, family obligations) as well as the needs of the pharmacy. For that reason, be sure to discuss the number of hours that you can work per day and per week so that you can fulfill the required number of experiential hours needed for your program. Once your preceptor has created the schedule, make a copy for yourself as well as one for your academic adviser. Any subsequent changes to your schedule must be approved by your preceptor and your externship coordinator.

Your coordinator will provide you with guidance on the completion of daily or weekly time sheets and their form of submission (either a paper or an electronic form). Your coordinator will also relay the options for making up missed time due to illness, vacation, or an emergency. Be aware that your time sheets must accurately reflect the time you have worked at the pharmacy (see the Workplace Wisdom box below) and must be signed by your preceptor and submitted to your externship coordinator either weekly or at the completion of your externship.

Finally, your preceptor will discuss the ramifications of habitual tardiness and distracted behaviors at work. Engaging in these behaviors reflects a poor work ethic and has a negative impact on your performance evaluations. Be aware that continuing these behaviors after warnings from your preceptor may result in a failing final grade or termination of your externship.

WORKPLACE WISDOM

Doctoring Time Sheets

Your time sheets must reflect an accurate, truthful account of your work hours at the pharmacy. If you were to claim hours you did not work during your employment, you likely would be terminated. If you were to forge hours you did not work during your externship, you likely would be terminated as well. These actions reflect dishonest, unethical behavior, which cannot be traits of a pharmacy technician.

Review Evaluation and Grading Parameters Typically, you will receive two performance evaluations: one midterm appraisal and one final appraisal. These evaluations are completed by your preceptor and reflect observations of your demonstrated competency in each learning objective. Both evaluations are conducted in a private setting.

During the midterm and final evaluations, your preceptor will provide you with feedback on practice areas in which you excel as well as areas that need continued development. These evaluations are similar to annual employee evaluations and should be used as a tool for continual improvement.

You or your preceptor will send a copy of your midterm and final evaluations to your externship coordinator. These evaluations, as well as related activities assigned by your coordinator, will factor in to your final grade for the term.

Participate in a Facility Orientation Before the start of your externship, your preceptor will conduct a facility orientation to explain the pharmacy's hours of operation, layout, and security. Your preceptor will also discuss areas for vehicle parking and storage of your personal belongings.

Practice Tip

During your facility orientation, you may be asked to sign a Code of Conduct, indicating your understanding of the behavior expectations for pharmacy personnel.

One important topic that your preceptor may cover during your orientation is the facility's **Policy and Procedures (P&P) manual**. The P&P manual discusses the policies and procedures that reflect federal and state laws governing pharmacy practice. The manual also outlines specific pharmacy procedures that allow the facility to run safely and efficiently. Additional topics in the P&P manual relate to pharmacy personnel, such as their roles; scope of practice; expected professional behaviors and disciplinary actions for failing to meet those expectations; dress code, including personal ID badges; and ethical responsibilities. Be sure that you study the facility's P&P manual so that your actions are aligned with the pharmacy's policies.

Your facility orientation also provides an opportunity for you to meet some of your pharmacy colleagues. Use this opportunity to create a good first impression with individuals by offering a friendly greeting and acknowledging that you are looking forward to working with them and learning from their expertise. These individuals will be invaluable resources to help you navigate your work responsibilities. They may also be assigned to train you in various areas of the pharmacy.

Self-Reflection:
Are You Ready to Work with Your Preceptor?

Read each statement. If you feel confident that you can say "yes" to that statement, place a check mark in the first column. For any unchecked statement, consider what steps you can take to improve in that area.

✔	Statement
	I know the role of my externship preceptor.
	I understand the importance of building a strong working relationship with my preceptor.
	I have considered what questions I would like to ask my preceptor before beginning my externship.
	I have prepared answers to questions I may be asked by my preceptor at our initial meeting.

Continues...

✔	Statement
	I am comfortable asking my preceptor questions about what I am expected to learn while participating in my externship.
	I understand that I am accountable for my attitude and behaviors during my externship.
	I understand the importance of constructive criticism by my preceptor and am open to it.
	I understand the practice areas that my preceptor will assess for my midterm and final evaluations.

8.6 Externship Practice

As mentioned earlier in this module, you may be assigned to one experiential rotation in a community pharmacy or institutional pharmacy, or you may need to fulfill two rotations. Regardless, your work performance will be measured by how well you achieve professional and technical competencies, or demonstrated proficiencies or skills in a specific area.

Professional competencies are universal to all practice sites and include good communication skills, ethical behavior, time management, multicultural awareness and cultural competence, professional appearance, and critical thinking and problem solving. These professional skills are assessed by your preceptor during your externship and are reflected on your midterm and final evaluations. Professional competencies are covered in the other eight modules of *Career Readiness & Externships: Soft Skills for Pharmacy Technicians* and, consequently, won't be specifically addressed here.

Technical competencies may be universal or specific to a community or an institutional pharmacy practice site. Your awareness and understanding of universal and specific technical competencies are critical to your daily responsibilities and your performance evaluations during your externship. Several of these technical competencies are addressed below.

Achieving Universal Technical Competencies

At the foundational level, pharmacies in all settings strive for the same goal: to safely and accurately dispense medications for patients. In many instances, the underlying processes are the same: keep medications in stock; enter prescriptions or medication orders; prepare the medications; and interact with customers, patients, and healthcare professionals. In addition to these foundational tasks, other competencies are universal to all pharmacy settings: adhere to federal and state laws and regulations, including scope of practice; know basic pharmacology; perform accurate pharmacy calculations; and implement proper medication safety practices. As a result, these competencies are worded in general terms on midterm and final externship evaluation forms.

Adhere to Federal and State Laws and Regulations To pass these competencies, an extern must follow all federal and state laws and regulations pertaining to pharmacy practice. Examples of these regulations include the completion of HIPAA training to ensure patient confidentiality; an adherence to the storage, handling, and dispensing of controlled substances; an understanding of the labeling of prescription medications; and an understanding of the scope of practice of pharmacy technicians. Be sure that you follow the policies and procedures of your school and your practice site. These policies and procedures are based on federal and state laws and regulations; therefore, your adherence to these protocols allows you to pass legal competencies with ease. (For more information on these competencies, refer to Module 7.)

Know Pharmacology An extern must demonstrate technical competencies in several areas of pharmacology. These competency areas include knowing the generic names and brand names of medications, drug classes, routes of administration, dosage formulations, indications for use, side effects and adverse effects, contraindications, and drug interactions. While memorization is the first level of knowing these pharmacology areas, knowledge of how medications cause their intended effects allows you to be a more effective pharmacy technician and be more confident in your externship responsibilities.

Perform Pharmacy Calculations Pharmacy calculations are a vitally important pharmacy technician responsibility. You are expected to have an understanding of basic mathematical operations (e.g., adding, subtracting, multiplying, and dividing of fractions as well as the proper use of decimals), a knowledge of Arabic number and Roman numeral systems, an ability to convert ratios and percentages, a knowledge of metric and household systems and the conversions within and between these systems, and an understanding of day's supply and quantity calculations. A consistent demonstration of accurate pharmacy calculations allows you to pass these technical competencies.

"To ensure medication safety, you must demonstrate deliberate, detail-oriented actions in your daily practices as an extern."

Implement Medication Safety Practices To ensure medication safety, you must demonstrate deliberate, detail-oriented actions in your daily practices as an extern. Technical competencies in this area include verifying and accurately filling prescriptions or medication orders, double-checking pharmacy calculations, checking labeling and packaging of medications, handling computer warning screens properly, and assisting in medication reconciliation and medication therapy management. Many of the processes and

Career Readiness & Externships: Soft Skills for Pharmacy Technicians

safeguards dictated by the policies and procedures of your pharmacy practice site ensure the highest level of safety in medication dispensing. Consequently, your adherence to these pharmacy protocols allows you to pass these technical competencies.

In addition, you should be familiar with several medication safety initiatives that alert you to the potential dangers of handling certain medications. These initiatives include the following resources from the Institute for Safe Medication Practices (ISMP):

- *List of Confused Drug Names*
- *List of Error-Prone Abbreviations, Symbols, and Dose Designations*
- *List of High-Alert Medications in Acute Care Settings*
- *List of High-Alert Medications in Community/Ambulatory Settings*

Achieving Technical Competencies Specific to Community Pharmacy Settings

In a community pharmacy setting, you will prepare prescriptions for dispensing directly to customers and initiate payment requests. You will also help to ensure that the pharmacy is stocked with sufficient quantities of required medications. Some of the technical competencies necessary to accomplish these goals include processing and dispensing prescriptions; using technology/informatics; implementing quality assurance practices; managing procurement, billing, reimbursement, and inventory of pharmacy supplies; and understanding insurance/billing practices.

Process and Dispense Prescriptions Competencies in this area involve assisting the pharmacist in collecting patient demographic information, including new patient intake and data entry; receiving and screening prescriptions for completion, accuracy, and authenticity; and preparing medications for dispensing, including selecting the correct medication, counting tablets and capsules, and labeling prescription vials. A large part of screening prescriptions is understanding the **signa**, or instructions for use. This understanding ensures proper calculation of both quantity and day's supply for a prescription, as well as additional instructions for use of the medication. A strong knowledge of medical abbreviations and terminology is necessary for this process.

Use Technology/Informatics Expected technical competencies in a community pharmacy include learning and navigating the pharmacy's software program. As mentioned earlier, this software provides a patient database and allows you to enter prescription information, print labels, and track medication inventory. To pass this competency, you must demonstrate consistent accuracy in entering patient and drug information. Other technology competencies you may encounter include the use of a pill-counting machine, bar-code scanning devices, and reconstitution devices.

Ensure Quality Assurance of Environment Quality assurance competencies you must demonstrate in a community pharmacy environment include monitoring the cleanliness of work areas; equipment, such as pill-counting machines; and nonsterile compounding work environments. In addition, you may be asked to calibrate digital scales to ensure accuracy and to monitor refrigerator and freezer temperatures at required intervals to ensure the quality, safety, and effectiveness of stored medications.

These monitoring activities are documented via log sheets. If these activities are assigned to you, make sure you fill out the appropriate log sheet consistently and accurately to pass this competency.

Manage Procurement and Inventory of Pharmacy Supplies In a community pharmacy, technical competencies include the initiation, verification, and billing for pharmacy goods and services. These competencies may require you to perform business-related calculations, such as overhead, gross and net profit, and markup.

Other technical competencies you may need to demonstrate relate to inventory management, such as receiving daily orders for restocking medications, verifying expiration dates of medications, returning medications to stock, handling product recalls, and reviewing medications in inventory quarterly.

Understand Insurance/Billing Procedures Insurance and billing competencies address your knowledge of medical insurance providers, patient insurance coverage for prescription drugs, prior authorization, and billing of medications. **Prior authorization** is a process that requires communication with a prescriber and an insurance provider to confirm medical necessity and ensure reimbursement for a medication or medical device before dispensing or sale. This insurance knowledge is a technical competency but is closely tied to a professional competency: your ability to provide clear communication and active listening in your interactions with customers and prescribers regarding prescription drug insurance.

Billing prescriptions involves adjudication. **Adjudication** is the process of determining how much of the cost of the prescription will be covered by the insurance company when processing an order. It may require communication with insurance companies to determine coverage on specific medications or for particular patients.

Achieving Technical Competencies Specific to Institutional Pharmacy Settings

In an institutional pharmacy setting, you will prepare medications for delivery to different units in the facility while ensuring that the equipment used is properly maintained and kept within appropriate operating ranges. Some of the technical competencies learned in this setting include processing medication orders; performing nonsterile and sterile compounding; using technology/informatics; implementing quality assurance practices; and managing procurement, billing, reimbursement, and inventory of pharmacy supplies.

Process Medication Orders Technical competencies in an institutional pharmacy involve processing medication orders rather than prescriptions. These orders are often submitted electronically by nursing units. Medication orders are typically written by physicians or other licensed prescribers in patients' charts, scanned by charge nurses on the hospital units, and sent to the pharmacy. These orders contain patient care directives and medications for patients during their hospital stay. If your institution allows pharmacy technicians to perform order-entry operations, you will identify what drugs and dosages have been ordered, enter them into the pharmacy software, create labels for each medication, and then fill the orders for delivery to nursing units.

To fill these orders, you may need to consult online drug databases that are available in an institutional setting, such as Micromedex or Lexicomp. You may also need to refer to printed drug reference materials, such as texts on injectable medications and pediatric dosing.

Perform Nonsterile and Sterile Compounding The processing of medication orders may require you to perform nonsterile or sterile compounding of medications. **Nonsterile compounding** is the preparation of a patient-specific medication or dosage form that is not commercially available. For example, you may need to reconstitute a powdered medication, create a suspension from a crushed tablet or capsule, or prepare a topical cream or ointment. Regardless of the task, you will follow a specific recipe, perform necessary calculations, and prepare the medication in a sanitized compounding space in the pharmacy. For these operations, specialized equipment—such as digital scales, ointment mills, and compounding slabs—may be used. Standards for nonsterile compounding are in the *United States Pharmacopeia* General Chapter <795>, more commonly referred to as *USP* <795>. Knowledge of *USP* <795> allows for efficient training of this technical competency during your externship program.

Sterile compounding is the dilution, mixing, reconstitution, or otherwise altering of various drugs or drug substances to create a sterile medication using **aseptic technique**. Sterile compounding procedures are performed by individuals who received special training, passed competency assessments, and—where applicable—achieved certification to compound sterile products for patient administration. Standards for sterile compounding are in *USP* General Chapter <797>, more commonly referred to as *USP* <797>. Knowledge of *USP* <797> allows for efficient training of this technical competency during your externship program.

Use Technology/Informatics Similar to a community pharmacy setting, expected technical competencies in an institutional pharmacy include learning and navigating the pharmacy's software program. Because many practitioners use an electronic health record, you have access to intake records and patient medical and medication histories, medication orders, and electronic medication administration records. Once you access the medication order, you can proceed with medication filling and distribution.

You may occasionally receive a handwritten medication order via personal delivery, fax, phone call, or pneumatic tube. Using the pharmacy's software program, you must input the medication order and have the information verified by a pharmacist. In other instances, you would be required to credit a patient's profile for unused orders to be returned to pharmacy stock. To pass the technical competency of navigating a pharmacy's software program, you must demonstrate an understanding of the different functions of the program.

In addition to learning a hospital pharmacy's software program, you are expected to learn and demonstrate your understanding of any specialized technology used in a given institutional setting. Examples of this technology include an automated dispensing cabinet, such as the commonly used Omnicell or Pyxis MedStation, or a medication inventory control system, such as Talyst or Pyxis C^{II}Safe. Newer devices, such as the Kit Check medication tray and cart management system, include radio-frequency identification (RFID) technology. These technical competencies are evaluated by your preceptor.

Ensure Quality Assurance of Environment In an institutional pharmacy, infection-control measures are critical to the health and safety of patients. The quality assurance policies in a facility are designed to monitor the mechanisms and processes that are used to prevent contamination of medications before they are dispensed, which includes storage requirements and preparation protocols.

You may be asked to monitor refrigerator and freezer temperatures at required intervals to ensure the quality, safety, and effectiveness of stored medications. You may also be tasked with completing log sheets for cleaning primary engineering controls, more commonly referred to as *hoods*; calibrating the compounder; and checking the expiration dates of medications. These technical competencies are components of your externship evaluations.

Manage Procurement, Billing, Reimbursement, and Inventory of Pharmacy Supplies Unlike a community pharmacy, an institutional pharmacy uses a single **drug formulary**, or a list of approved drugs for use in the facility. This list is based on the recommendations of the hospital's Pharmacy and Therapeutics (P&T) Committee. The P&T Committee considers several factors when creating a drug formulary: generic drug preferences, effectiveness of drugs, hospital budgets, and insurance reimbursements. To order medications for the pharmacy, you may work with pharmaceutical sales representatives to receive bids and purchase contracts. Once the medications are received at the pharmacy, you may check the order against the wholesaler's or manufacturer's receipt and store the medications in inventory. Placing the daily order of medications in inventory as well as working with and shadowing the buyer (a specialized role held commonly by a pharmacy technician) satisfy these technical competencies in an institutional pharmacy setting.

Inventory management competencies involve filling unit-dose and emergency crash carts for patient care units; processing the returned unit-dose carts; stocking the automated central pharmacy and floor stock dispensing units; monitoring inventory and narcotic control in both the pharmacy and nursing units; verifying the expiration dates of medications, including the expiration dates of drugs on emergency crash carts; returning medications to stock; and handling product recalls.

8.7 Module Summary

Completing a pharmacy technician externship provides you with many benefits: an assessment of your knowledge and skills, an opportunity for real-world pharmacy practice, a training experience in pharmacy software programs, and an opportunity for mentorship and networking. Your participation in an externship also provides the practice site with many benefits, such as an additional staff member to help with operations.

You must complete several basic and program-specific externship requirements. Basic externship requirements include submitting personal ID, educational documents, and registration/certification documents as appropriate. In addition, if your academic program is ASHP/ACPE-accredited, you must fulfill the pharmacy education and training standards of these organizations. These standards dictate the number of health-related curriculum hours and the specific educational modality of these hours—didactic, simulated, and experiential. Program-specific externship requirements include knowledge of the learning objectives, extern responsibilities, related externship assignments, required hours, and federal and state pharmacy laws and regulations.

To participate in an externship, you must undergo a pre-externship health screening. This screening includes a physical exam, an immunization update, a drug-screening test, and a criminal background check. These health-screening components have specific, individual requirements that must be met. Failure to meet these requirements prohibits you from participating in a pharmacy technician externship.

You are assigned a specific practice site and a preceptor who guides you through the externship experience. At the initial meeting, your preceptor discusses the role of a preceptor and the professional relationship that exists between a preceptor and an extern. In addition, your preceptor addresses your rotation requirements, work schedule, midterm and final evaluations, grading parameters, and expected professional and technical competencies of your externship.

Technical competencies may be universal or specific to a community or an institutional pharmacy practice site. Universal technical competencies include adherence to federal and state laws and regulations, including scope of practice; knowledge of pharmacology; performance of accurate pharmacy calculations; and implementation of medication safety practices. Specific technical competencies associated with community pharmacies include processing and dispensing prescriptions, using pharmacy software programs and other technology, implementing environmental quality assurance standards, procuring and conducting inventory of pharmacy supplies, and conducting insurance and billing procedures. Specific technical competencies related to institutional pharmacies include processing medication orders; executing nonsterile and sterile compounding; using pharmacy software programs and other technology; implementing environmental quality assurance standards; and managing procurement, billing, reimbursement, and inventory of pharmacy supplies.

 The online course includes additional review and assessment resources.

Career Readiness, Planning, & Management

LEARNING OBJECTIVES

1 Describe the career competencies identified by the National Association of Colleges and Employers (NACE). (Section 9.1)

2 Understand the importance of pharmacy technician certification to your career readiness. (Section 9.2)

3 Identify the two types of pharmacy technician certification exams: Pharmacy Technician Certification Exam (PTCE) and Exam for the Certification of Pharmacy Technicians (ExCPT). (Section 9.2)

4 Explore your career options by gathering information from career services, online research, career fairs, and professional mentors. (Section 9.2)

5 Describe the steps to take in a job search, including a check of your online presence and the creation of a résumé, cover letter, career portfolio, and job application. (Section 9.3)

6 Prepare for a job interview by researching the hiring company, anticipating the type of interview, reviewing common interview questions, and practicing your interviewing skills. (Section 9.3)

7 Conduct a successful job interview by making a good first impression, staying focused and honest in your responses, and posing questions to the interviewer. (Section 9.4)

8 Establish a career path by setting short-term and long-term goals, joining professional organizations and networking, and participating in continuing and advanced educational opportunities. (Section 9.5)

To view the *ASHP/ACPE Accreditation Standards* addressed in this chapter, refer to Appendix A.

The successful completion of your academic/training program and externship marks the end of one journey and the beginning of another journey: launching your professional career. Just as your postsecondary education began with a vision, careful planning and preparation, and an established route to achieve that vision, so too does a professional career journey.

This module walks you through each stage of your professional career journey—from career readiness through career management—and provides the steps you need to take in each stage. Some of the topics addressed include achieving pharmacy technician certification, exploring career options, reviewing your online presence and social media accounts, creating a résumé and cover letter, preparing for a job interview, and setting career goals.

9.1 Career Readiness

According to the National Association of Colleges and Employers (NACE), **career readiness** is "the attainment and demonstration of requisite competencies that broadly prepare college graduates for a successful transition into the workplace." Now that you are making that transition, you should be aware of these career competencies, or employability skills, that an employer is seeking in a potential job candidate. Although you have already attained many of these competencies during your academic program, research has shown that you likely need additional employability skills training to achieve workplace excellence and overall career success.

Understanding Career Competencies

NACE outlines the **career competencies** that employers want in their job candidates. These competencies address the following areas:

- *Critical thinking/problem solving:* Exercise sound reasoning to analyze issues, make decisions, and overcome obstacles
- *Oral/written communications:* Articulate thoughts and ideas clearly and effectively in written and oral communications to individuals inside and outside of a company or facility
- *Teamwork/collaboration:* Build collaborative relationships with colleagues, vendors, customers, or patients representing diverse cultures, races, ages, genders, religions, lifestyles, and viewpoints
- *Digital technology:* Use existing digital technologies ethically and efficiently to solve problems, complete tasks, and accomplish goals
- *Leadership:* Leverage the strengths of others to achieve common goals
- *Professionalism/work ethic:* Demonstrate personal accountability, an effective work ethic (punctuality, productivity, and time management), and a professional image

- *Global/intercultural fluency:* Value, respect, and learn from diverse cultures, races, ages, genders, sexual orientations, and religions
- *Career management:* Identify and articulate your skills, strengths, knowledge, and experiences relevant to the position desired and career goals; identify areas necessary for professional growth

You will find information on all NACE career competencies in the modules of *Career Readiness & Externships: Soft Skills for Pharmacy Technicians*. This module focuses on career management, or the ability to articulate your knowledge, skills, and experience related to a desired position; explore career options; understand the steps needed to pursue job opportunities; and identify areas for potential career growth.

Gaining Self-Awareness

Launching a professional career that leads to personal fulfillment and success begins with self-awareness. You need to identify who you are, what skills you have acquired, and what you want in your career and personal life. Once you have identified those qualities, you can then determine what you can offer to a potential employer. To help you gauge your self-awareness, refer to the Self-Reflection activity below.

 Self-Reflection:
How Well Do You Know Yourself?

Read each statement. If you feel confident that you can say "yes" to that statement, place a check mark in the first column. For any unchecked statement, consider what steps you can take to gain self-awareness in that area.

✔	Statement
	I know my priorities for my career.
	I know what type of position best suits my personality, skills, and interests.
	I recognize the personality traits and skill sets that are my strengths.
	I recognize the personality traits and skill sets that are my weaknesses.
	I have a set of principles that guides my career decisions.
	I can describe my ideal supervisor.
	I can describe my ideal work environment.
	I can describe my ideal coworkers.
	I know the type of lifestyle I want.
	I have my own definition of personal success.
	I can describe my work ethic.

9.2 Career Planning

Embarking on a successful professional career requires you to plan. Achieving your pharmacy technician national certification is a great first step in making yourself marketable to a pharmacy. It conveys to an employer a high level of commitment and competency as a pharmacy technician.

Other possible career-planning steps you can take include visiting the career services department at your institution, conducting online research, attending a career fair, or working with a recruiter. You may also want to seek wisdom and guidance from a professional mentor.

Achieving Pharmacy Technician National Certification

Now that you have completed your educational/training requirements, the first step in your career journey may be the pursuit of pharmacy technician national certification. **Certification** is the process by which a nongovernmental association grants recognition to an individual who has met certain predetermined qualifications specified by that profession. To achieve the designation of **certified pharmacy technician (CPhT)**, you must pass a national certification examination. Two pharmacy technician certification exams are offered in the United States: the Pharmacy Technician Certification Exam (PTCE) and the Exam for the Certification of Pharmacy Technicians (ExCPT). Once you achieve certification, you are required to earn continuing education credits to renew your certification.

Prepare for the Pharmacy Technician Certification Exam The **Pharmacy Technician Certification Exam (PTCE)**, offered by the **Pharmacy Technician Certification Board (PTCB)**, is the most widely used exam and is accepted by the boards of pharmacy in all 50 states and in the District of Columbia. As of December 31, 2018, the PTCB granted more than 676,000 pharmacy technician certifications to individuals who passed the PTCE.

The PTCE is a multiple-choice exam containing 90 questions—80 of which are scored. The remaining 10 questions are not scored but rather are tested for future inclusion into the exam. You will take the exam on a computer located at a testing center, and you will have two hours to complete the exam.

To learn more about the PTCE, visit the PTCB website at https://SSPharm.ParadigmEducation.com/PTCB. Once there, you will find detailed information on the following topics related to the certification exam:

- eligibility requirements
- list of the knowledge domains tested, which can be used as a study guide
- procedures for registering and taking the exam
- scoring criteria for passing the exam
- process for renewal of certification

The PTCB website also has a downloadable publication for test applicants titled *Certification Guidelines and Requirements: A Candidate Guidebook.* This publication offers information about all aspects of PTCB certification for pharmacy technicians and includes information about the new Certified Compounded Sterile Preparation Technician (CSPT) exam (see the Workplace Wisdom feature box below).

WORKPLACE WISDOM

SCAT Certification

In 2018, the PTCB launched the first national pharmacy technician certification exam for sterile compounding and aseptic technique (SCAT). Passing this advanced exam grants the credential of Certified Compounded Sterile Preparation Technician (CSPT). While many training programs have granted certificates for the preparation of sterile products, this PTCB certification requires continuing education and annual renewal to remain active. To be eligible to apply for the CSPT exam, a pharmacy technician must:

- be a CPhT through the PTCB and be in good standing

- have completed a PTCB-recognized sterile compounding education/training program plus one year of continuous, full-time, compounded sterile preparation work experience or three years of continuous, full-time, compounded sterile preparation work experience

Therefore, if your long-term career goal is to achieve sterile compounding and aseptic technique certification, you may want to consider sitting for the PTCE, which is the only acceptable prerequisite exam for this advanced certification.

Prepare for the Exam for the Certification of Pharmacy Technicians The **Exam for the Certification of Pharmacy Technicians (ExCPT)**, offered by the **National Healthcareer Association (NHA)**, is currently accepted by a portion of the state boards of pharmacy. As of December 31, 2018, the NHA granted more than 23,000 pharmacy technician certifications to individuals who passed the ExCPT.

The ExCPT is a multiple-choice exam containing 120 questions—100 of which are scored. The remaining 20 questions are considered pretest questions and are not scored. You will take the exam on a computer located at a testing center, and you will have 2 hours and 10 minutes to complete the exam.

To learn more about the ExCPT, visit the NHA website at https://SSPharm.ParadigmEducation.com/NHA. Once there, you will find detailed information on the following topics:

- eligibility requirements
- list of the knowledge domains tested (Test Plan), which can be used as a study guide
- procedures for registering and taking the exam
- scoring criteria for passing the exam
- process for renewal of certification

In addition to the downloadable Test Plan, NHA offers additional study materials to prepare for the ExCPT exam.

Renewing Pharmacy Technician National Certification

Whether you take the PTCE or the ExCPT, you are required to renew your national certification within a specified time frame. The renewal process involves paying a fee and submitting a required number of continuing education credits to the certifying body. This process is outlined in the guidebooks for the PTCE and the ExCPT. In addition, the guidebooks outline the protocol that must be followed if you fail to renew your certification within the allotted period.

Participate in Continuing Education **Continuing education (CE)** is a course of study or a set of learning activities that enables participants to maintain or enhance their knowledge or skills in a professional field after they have left their formal education. Participation in these learning activities allows individuals to earn **continuing education (CE) credits** or **continuing education units (CEUs)**. CEs or CEUs are required when renewing your pharmacy technician certification. Although these credits can be earned through various means, the most common delivery method is online courses. When taking an online CE course, you typically watch or read material on a given subject in pharmacy, such as medication safety, sterile compounding, law, etc. Once you have reviewed the material, you then take a quiz to verify your understanding of the content. If you pass the quiz, you receive the credit for the course.

CEs or CEUs are measured in credit hours—for example, 1.0 hour of CE. The designated number is equivalent to how many hours it should take to review the material presented. Typically, CEs or CEUs are available as 1.0 to 3.0 hours of CE credit, depending on the course content. Both the PTCE and the ExCPT require a certain number of CEs for certification renewal, and a portion of those credit hours must be in a specific content area, such as medication safety or law. To review the specific CE requirements for the PTCE and the ExCPT, visit their respective websites.

Accreditation and CEs **Accreditation** is the process by which an organization or a facility (university or college) has met the quality standards of a specific profession or industry. Consequently, a CE issued by an accredited organization is considered valid and acceptable for certification renewal. The **Accreditation Council for Pharmacy Education (ACPE)** is the organization that accredits colleges of pharmacy and CEs for both pharmacists and pharmacy technicians. An accredited CE has an ACPE number in the description of the course. This number looks similar to a National Drug Code (NDC) number for a medication; however, the letter "P" or the letter "T" appears at the end of the number. This letter designates whether the CE content is specific to pharmacists (P) or technicians (T). An example of an ACPE number for pharmacy technicians is 0430-0000-18-015-H02-T.

Track CE Credits To keep track of your CE credits, or access and print transcripts of your CE credits for license renewal or for state board requirements, you will use an online database that stores and authenticates your information. This database, known as *CPE Monitor*, is a collaborative service of ACPE, ACPE providers, and the **National Association of Boards of Pharmacy (NABP)**. To use this service, create a free account. You will be assigned a unique CPE Monitor identification number. Remember this number because you may be asked to give this number when completing an online CE course.

Exploring Career Options

There are many career options available to pharmacy technicians. You may want to work in a community pharmacy because you enjoy patient contact or a mail-order pharmacy because you like to work independently. Perhaps your calling is an institutional pharmacy where you can work with medication distribution systems, such as a unit-dose cart or an automated floor stock system.

To find a pharmacy technician position that is best suited for you, consider your personal qualities, interests, education, and skill sets. You should arm yourself with as much information as possible regarding the various career paths available to pharmacy technicians. Spend time using your career services department, researching different positions, attending career fairs, and enlisting help from a professional mentor.

Enlist Help from Career Services Almost every educational institution has a **career services department**. The primary responsibility of this department is to provide current students and graduates with information on the knowledge and skills needed to secure a position in their chosen field. The department assists with résumé writing, interview preparation, and job leads. Make sure to take the initiative to meet with the department regarding your career options.

Research Pharmacy Technician Positions Performing online research into pharmacy technician positions that interest you is a great way to focus your job search. The Bureau of Labor Statistics provides a general overview of the roles and responsibilities of pharmacy technicians in its *Occupational Outlook Handbook* accessed at https://SSPharm.ParadigmEducation.com/OOH. The *Handbook* lists national pay averages, required education/training, scope of work, number of jobs, and job outlook.

To find more specific information on available pharmacy technician openings in your state, region, city, or town, visit job-search websites, such as Indeed (https://SSPharm.ParadigmEducation.com/Indeed) or Monster (https://SSPharm.ParadigmEducation.com/Monster). These sites list all pharmacy technician positions posted in a particular area and include a job description for each opening.

To organize the information that you gather in your research, create a table that provides a snapshot of pertinent information about each pharmacy technician position. Record your comments regarding what you like (pros) and don't like (cons) about each position based on the information you find (see Table 9.1).

Attend Career Fairs A **career fair** is a gathering of representatives from various companies who want to recruit new employees for their facilities. These representatives may accept job applications or résumés from attendees, schedule follow-up interviews, or even conduct interviews at the event. Many vocational colleges host their own career fairs and invite companies tailored to the programs they offer.

If you attend a career fair, approach the event as you would a job interview: Bring all of your materials (résumé, transcripts, etc.), dress for success, and be prepared to make a great first impression. If you are researching career fairs not hosted by your educational institution, be sure to search for "pharmacy technician career fairs." The majority of community career fairs are geared toward industries unrelated to health care.

Use Recruiting Companies **Recruiting companies**, also known as *employment agencies*, can also be a resource in your career search. These companies are paid by employers to help them fill their staffing needs. Many of these companies have job boards similar to Indeed or Monster that you can view. If you are interested in a position, you can submit an online job application. As with career fairs, make sure to search for pharmacy-specific recruiters who specialize in pharmacist and pharmacy technician employment opportunities.

Find a Professional Mentor A **professional mentor** is an individual who can provide you with guidance, advice, and support during your career search and professional experience. Therefore, this individual should have knowledge and expertise in the pharmacy setting. When looking for a professional

Table 9.1 Pharmacy Technician Positions

Position	Prerequisites for Employment	Responsibilities	Pros	Cons
Hospital purchasing agent	• State license • One year of hospital experience • National certification	• Maintains inventory, budget, and back orders • Receives inventory supplies	• Autonomy • Inventory management • Increased responsibility	• Budget accountability • Back orders
Call center technician	• State trainee license, regular license, or national certification • Familiarity with Microsoft Office • Bilingual proficiency a plus • Customer service experience a plus	• Communicates with customers via phone, email, online chat, and social media • Maintains customer profile in database • Provides feedback on call issues	• Desk job (less standing) • Data entry • Critical thinking practice • Customer service experience	• Sedentary work environment (sitting too much) • Disgruntled customer interactions
Community pharmacy technician	• Fluency in English (reading, writing, and speaking) • National certification and/or state-required certification/registration • Flexible schedule • Good math skills preferred • Good computer skills preferred	• Enters patient and drug information into computer • Fills prescriptions • Handles currency • Answers telephone and addresses inquiries • Processes insurance claims • Assists with inventory duties	• Face-to-face patient interactions • Variety of job duties • Customer service interactions • No sterile compounding	• Insurance claim handling • Disgruntled customer interactions

mentor, consider a former graduate or instructor from your academic/ training program, your former preceptor, or a former colleague from your externship. You may also know someone who influenced you in entering the pharmacy technician field. Any of these individuals can provide you with insight on career options, job searches, and workplace wisdom.

Asking someone to be a mentor is asking that person to invest time and energy into your success. Therefore, seek a mentor with qualities that will allow the relationship to succeed, such as an individual who has:

- forged a comfortable relationship with you
- earned your respect

- garnered the respect of colleagues and peers in the pharmacy profession
- demonstrated effective communication skills
- exhibited a willingness to provide constructive feedback
- achieved the same goal or a similar goal to the one you are attempting to achieve
- shown a genuine interest in your success

After you have identified a potential mentor, contact that individual and explain why you are seeking that individual's professional guidance in your career search. If the individual agrees to help you, arrange a meeting to discuss different career paths you are interested in pursuing. Prepare for your meeting by narrowing your list of possible career options and formulating specific questions about these positions. Consider your mentor's feedback and suggestions for next steps as you start your career journey.

> ### Think It Through: Finding a Professional Mentor
> What individuals have had an influence on your pharmacy technician coursework or experiential training? Brainstorm a short list of potential individuals you might ask to be your professional mentor.

9.3 Job-Search Preparation

Now that you have devoted time to career readiness and have narrowed down your career options, you need to prepare for the job search. This preparation includes checking your online presence, reviewing your social media accounts, writing an effective résumé, composing a cover letter, assembling a career portfolio, completing a job application, and preparing for a job interview.

Checking Your Online Presence

Before your first job interview, you should check your **online presence** by entering your name into a search engine, such as Google. It also helps to enter your city of residence, such as "John Doe Los Angeles." Review both website listings and the image search to see what results are returned.

The goal of this search is to make sure that nothing is visible that might give the wrong impression of you to a potential employer. This "scrubbing" is useful, as there may be a picture of you that conveys an image that you don't want associated with your professional career. Many image results will invariably lead back to any articles about you, as well as any social media accounts you may have.

Reviewing Your Social Media Accounts

According to a 2017 online survey conducted by the Harris Poll for CareerBuilder, 70% of employers review the social media accounts of job applicants. This common practice provides them with a profile of the applicant, including the individual's personality, interests, and activities. With that in mind, reviewing your social media accounts is an important step to take before conducting a job search.

When reviewing your social media accounts, consider the following recommendations:

- Remove any posts that you would not want a prospective employer to see.
- Check for comments that others would interpret as racist, sexist, or discriminatory.
- Remove or untag photos that depict you in an unfavorable light.
- Review your page and comments from your friends and remove any items that are inappropriate.
- Check the apps on your profile to see if they reflect you in a favorable light.
- Review the names of groups in which you belong to check their appropriateness.
- Review privacy settings to control what viewers outside of your social group can see.

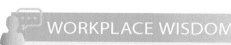

WORKPLACE WISDOM

Incognito Online Search
To view what an individual can see when your name is entered into a search engine, sign out of any browser profile and perform the search under "incognito mode" in Chrome. This anonymous setting provides results that are not based on your own search history algorithms and more accurately reflect what an employer might see in an online search.

EXPAND YOUR KNOWLEDGE

Social Media Matters
Hiring managers offer various reasons why they review the social media accounts of job applicants. The statistics below provide you with insight as to how your social media image has an effect on your professional career.

- Sixty-five percent said they use social media to investigate whether a candidate presents a professional image.
- Fifty-one percent said they use social media to see whether a job applicant would be a good fit for the company.

- Forty-five percent said they use social media to learn additional information about an applicant's qualifications.
- Thirty-five percent said they use social media to determine if an applicant is well-rounded.
- Twelve percent said they use social media to determine if there is a reason not to hire an applicant.

Building a Résumé

Work Wise

Do not use too many colors or graphics in the design of your résumé. A résumé that is too busy may decrease your chance of selection by an employer. In addition, these design elements may not transfer legibly in an online job application.

You may be surprised to hear that an employer spends 30 seconds or less reviewing an individual's résumé and determining whether to interview a job applicant. In light of that statistic, a well-written résumé can make the difference between securing an interview or receiving a rejection letter from a company or facility. Consider your résumé as an opportunity to create a favorable first impression with an employer. Consequently, it must have an engaging, easy-to-read format; accurate, concise content; and correct spelling, punctuation, capitalization, and grammar.

Select a Résumé Format Typically, a résumé follows one of three formats: chronological, skills-based, or a combination that is both chronological and skills-based. Choose a format that best suits your information.

Chronological Format Most individuals use a chronological format when crafting a résumé (see Figure 9.1). A **chronological résumé** lists your education and work experience starting with your current or most recent information listed first. This résumé format works well if you are a new entrant to the job market or if you have no gaps in your work history. A chronological format is also advantageous if you are completing an online job application because a computer can read and place the information in the correct areas of the application.

Figure 9.1 Chronological Résumé

The Work Experience portion of a chronological résumé traces your work history in reverse order (present to past).

Mirabel Le

555-555-5555

Mirabel.Le@ParadigmEducation.com

Job Objective

To be hired as a pharmacy technician in a community pharmacy after I graduate from college.

Work Experience

Walgreens Pharmacy, Las Vegas, NV—*Pharmacy Technician Extern*, March 2021

- Filled prescription orders for a 600-prescription-per-day pharmacy
- Assisted patients with receiving their prescriptions
- Performed insurance claim process
- Used QS1 pharmacy database program

El Portal Luggage, Las Vegas, NV—*Retail Associate*, January 2021 to Present

- Handled purchases and returns for customers
- Successfully assisted customers with product selections
- Managed inventory, including ordering and restocking of merchandise
- Assisted in setup of store displays

McDonalds, Las Vegas, NV—*Team Member*, June 2020 to December 2020

- Maintained high standards of customer service during high-volume operations

---

Skills-Based Format Another type of résumé uses a skills-based format (see Figure 9.2). A **skills–based résumé** groups your skills and experiences together rather than focusing on specific positions and dates. This résumé format works well for individuals who have gaps in their work history or have a short work history. A skills–based résumé also is a good choice if you are changing careers and do not have relevant work experience. Another advantage to this format is that you can tailor your résumé to match the skills noted in the job description.

Figure 9.2 Skills-Based Résumé

A skills-based résumé highlights your skill sets for an employer.

Mirabel Le

555-555-5555

Mirabel.Le@ParadigmEducation.com

Job Objective

Seeking employment as a pharmacy technician that will leverage my customer service skills and vocational training in an exciting community pharmacy environment

Skills Summary

Accuracy: experience working with cash drawers and ordering systems that required a high degree of accuracy

Effective communication skills: good written and verbal communication skills in one-on-one interactions and collaborative tasks; typing speed of 65 words per minute

Computer savviness: proficiency in both Windows and Mac operating systems and software; familiarity with pharmacy database software and its applications

Flexibility/dependability: ability to work long hours on days, evenings, and weekends; willingness to adapt to changing situations, including working at different pharmacy branches; access to reliable transportation

Strong work ethic: good time management; diligence in pharmacy-related tasks; professionalism

Work Experience

Walgreens Pharmacy, Las Vegas, NV—*Pharmacy Technician Extern*, March 2021

El Portal Luggage, Las Vegas, NV—*Retail Associate*, January 2021 to Present

McDonalds, Las Vegas, NV—*Team Member*, June 2020 to December 2020

Education

MyTown Career College, Spring 2020

Pharmacy Technician Diploma

Awards

- Perfect Attendance 8 of 12 terms at MyTown Career College
- Sales Award, Fourth Quarter, El Portal Luggage

Combination Format A third type of résumé uses a combination format (see Figure 9.3). A **combination résumé** merges some elements of a chronological résumé and some elements of a skills-based résumé. The first part of this type of résumé summarizes your relevant qualifications, skill sets, and experience. The second part provides a chronological framework of your work experience. A combination résumé works well if you are changing careers because its format highlights your stable employment as well as your skills.

Figure 9.3 Combination Résumé

A combination résumé offers a list of your skill sets and a detailed work history.

Mirabel Le

555-555-5555

Mirabel.Le@ParadigmEducation.com

Professional Profile

- **Project Execution**—Helped implement new point-of-sale and inventory tracking system, becoming versed in computer software upgrades and transitions
- **Communication**—Communicated with customers regularly, meeting monthly sales quotas for merchandise; bilingual in Spanish and English
- **Teamwork**—Worked effectively and efficiently with both coworkers and supervisors; received praise for teamwork on quarterly evaluation
- **Awards**—Maintained perfect attendance for 8 out of 12 terms during vocational training; received best sales member for fourth quarter

Skills Summary

- Good written and verbal communication skills
- Typing speed of 65 words per minute
- Familiar with pharmacy database software and its applications
- Ability to work days, evenings, and weekends
- Own reliable transportation and can commute to different pharmacy branches as necessary
- Ability to work long hours, maintain continuing education, and adapt to changing situations

Work Experience

El Portal Luggage, Las Vegas, NV—*Retail Associate*, January 2021 to Present

McDonalds, Las Vegas, NV—*Team Member*, June 2020 to December 2020

Education

MyTown Career College, Spring 2020

Pharmacy Technician Diploma

Externship Experience

Walgreens Pharmacy, Las Vegas, NV, March 2021

Assemble Your Résumé Components No matter the format, a résumé has six key components and one optional component. These components are typically presented in this order:

- personal/contact information
- job objective
- skills summary
- work experience
- education/certifications/licensures
- awards
- references (optional)

To determine the information that belongs in each component, refer to the sections below.

Personal/Contact Information Your personal/contact information should include your full name, your personal (not company) email address, and your telephone number. Make sure that your voicemail message and your personal email address are professional and appropriate.

Job Objective A **job objective** is a brief statement (one or two sentences) that indicates your desire to be hired and to find a position that suits your skill sets. For example, you may want to begin your job objective by stating "Secure (or obtain) a position with . . ." or "Begin working with a facility that. . . ." Then complete your statement by specifying the type of position you are looking for in your job search. For example, a job objective for a pharmacy technician position might be stated as follows: "To secure a pharmacy technician position in a community pharmacy where I can utilize my education/training and my organization, teamwork, and customer service skills."

Keep in mind these two rules when creating a job objective: The statement should be tailored to the position that you are seeking, and it should include some of the key words from the job description. If your job application and résumé are submitted online, the inclusion of these key words is especially critical. Many employers use an **applicant tracking system (ATS)** that flags key words from the job description in your submitted application and résumé. Consequently, documents that contain many flags are recommended to hiring managers for review. (See the Expand Your Knowledge feature box on the next page for more information on applicant tracking systems.)

Skills Summary Consider the skill sets that you have acquired in your education, training, and work experience. These skills should be presented

Practice Tip

Be sure that your personal email address is professional and consists of your first and last name.

Applicant Tracking System

An applicant tracking system (ATS) is a type of software that employers may use to screen potential job candidates. This program scans résumés submitted online for key words related to the job description and filters out the most relevant ones, which then are forwarded to the hiring manager. If this software is used by a hiring company and your submitted job application and résumé do not fit its screening algorithm, your documents may never be seen by a hiring manager.

Below are some tips to help ensure your résumé makes it past the initial ATS screening:

- Incorporate key words from the job description in your application and résumé.
- Use a common font and simple design in your résumé so that it can be read by the ATS.
- Spell out words rather than use abbreviations; for example, use "certified pharmacy technician" rather than "CPhT" in your résumé.

in the skills summary component of your résumé. You may want to address two skill categories:

- soft skills, such as demonstrated adaptability, teamwork, and problem-solving skills; good organizational skills; advanced pharmacy calculations skills; strong work ethic; good communication skills, including fluency in Spanish; etc.
- task-related skills, such as computer technology (e.g., proficiency in QS1 or Guardian Rx pharmacy databases); pharmacy technology (e.g., operational knowledge of Parata Max automated dispensing system or Pyxis, bar-code technology); inventory management; typing speed; etc.

Work Experience Each job in this component should be listed in reverse chronological order. The information should include the name of the company or facility, your job title, your hire date (month and year) and exit date (month and year), and several bulleted points that briefly summarize your job responsibilities. Because this information is typically the largest section of your résumé as well as a key component of your job candidacy, format the information to ensure readability and understanding. Consider using type treatments (such as boldface, italic, underlining, etc.) to set off certain items of information.

Education/Certifications/Licensures This résumé component should provide a summary of your education in reverse chronological order. This list should begin with your most recent postsecondary degree and end with your high school diploma. Each entry should include the following elements:

- name and location of the institution
- graduation date or expected graduation date
- name of your degree or area of specialization

In addition, you should state any certifications or licensures that you have achieved on your résumé. List each certification or licensure in reverse chronological order and include only those items that are directly related to the job opening. Each certification or licensure should provide the following information:

- name of the certification or licensure
- name of the certifying or licensing body
- date obtained and any expiration date
- state affiliation

Be sure to write out the full name of the certification or licensure followed by its acronym or abbreviation. For example, you should state "certified pharmacy technician (CPhT)" rather than simply "CPhT" on your résumé.

Awards In this résumé component, you should list any academic, externship, business, or employment awards you have received. Provide the name of the award, the name of the organization that bestowed the award, a brief description of the significance of the award, and the date you received the award.

References You may choose to include a list of references on your résumé. **References** are individuals who can attest to your character, education/training, skills, and work habits as well as your suitability for a job opening. When asking individuals to serve as references in your job search, consider people from various sectors of your life, such as education (instructors, preceptors, or colleagues); work experience (supervisors, department heads, or colleagues); and organizations (professional mentors, clergy, or volunteers).

If you do not want a list of references on your résumé, include the title of the component ("References") and state "References available on request" underneath the title. You should have copies of these references in your career portfolio. (For additional information on career portfolios, see the section titled "Assembling a Career Portfolio" later in this module.)

Practice Tip

Do not put any individuals on your reference list without first asking them for permission to do so.

Writing a Cover Letter

A **cover letter** typically accompanies a job application and is an opportunity for you (the job applicant) to introduce yourself to a potential employer, summarize your relevant qualifications, and request a meeting with the employer. This letter also showcases your ability to express yourself clearly and concisely and use proper writing conventions (grammar, spelling, punctuation, and capitalization). For that reason, you should spend some time creating a letter that creates a great first impression for a potential employer.

A cover letter should be brief (one page) and include five specific sections: header, salutation, introduction, body, and conclusion (see Figure 9.4). Keep your audience in mind when you write a cover letter. Be sure to highlight your qual-

Practice Tip

Several cover letter templates are available online and can help you format the letter. Two online templates can be found at the following locations: https://SSPharm.ParadigmEducation.com/CoverLetterTemplates and https://SSPharm.ParadigmEducation.com/MicrosoftTemplates.

ifications that align with the job description and include key words from that description in your cover letter. If you are submitting an online job application, you can copy and paste your cover letter directly into the application, or you can compose your cover letter directly in the available form field.

Figure 9.4 Cover Letter

A cover letter is your first opportunity to market yourself as the best candidate for a job opening.

Mirabel Le

555-555-5555

Mirabel.Le@ParadigmEducation.com

June 15, 2021

Bianca Solovar, PharmD

All City Pharmacy

1234 Broadway Street

Hometown, NV 12345

Dear Dr. Solovar:

I am writing regarding your job posting for a pharmacy technician at All City Pharmacy that was featured on Indeed.com. As you can see from my enclosed résumé, I have a diploma in pharmacy technology from MyTown Career College and achieved a 3.5 GPA in my academic program. My externship was in a community pharmacy, where I had real-world experience in day-to-day pharmacy operations, including production, insurance verification, and patient interactions. In addition to this externship, I have worked as a retail associate, which further enhanced my customer service skills. I take pride in performing professionally in a busy setting.

The education I have received and the roles that I have filled reflect my commitment to personal and professional excellence as a pharmacy technician. I would welcome the opportunity to speak with you about my qualifications. Thank you for your consideration, and I look forward to hearing from you soon.

Sincerely,

Mirabel Le, CPhT

Create a Header Similar to the format of a business letter, a header in a cover letter appears in the upper left section of the page and contains the date (month, day, and year); recipient's name; recipient's professional title; name of the company or facility; and business address of the company or facility. Oftentimes, you will not have the recipient's name and professional title to include in the header. In this situation, you should use a generic title for the recipient, such as "Human Resources Manager," "Hiring Manager," or "Hiring Recruiter."

Insert a Salutation A salutation appears after the header. If you know the name of the recipient, you should use a title of address followed by the recipient's last name:

- Dear Mr. Brasheres
- Dear Ms. Thao
- Dear Professor Reed
- Dear Dr. Singh

If you don't know the name of the recipient, you should use a generic salutation:

- To Whom It May Concern
- Dear Human Resources Manager
- Dear Hiring Manager

A colon is commonly used after a cover letter salutation because it denotes the formality of the correspondence. A comma is reserved to follow the salutation of a personal letter, which is an informal correspondence.

Compose an Introduction The introduction of your cover letter should be brief (a four- to six-sentence paragraph) and should capture the recipient's attention, express a little of your personality, and reveal your strong desire to be considered for the job opening. Consequently, the introduction should address the following questions:

- Who are you?
- What is the position you desire?
- Where did you learn about the position?
- Why do you want this position?

Develop a Body Section The body section of your cover letter should address how you can contribute to the company or facility. This section should be one or two paragraphs and should summarize your qualifications for the job opening. Your qualifications might include references to your education, training, work experience, or work habits that align with this job opening. The intent here is to highlight the assets that make you a good candidate for the position.

Practice Tip

When writing a cover letter, be sure that you are not restating your résumé but rather highlighting a few of your qualifications.

Write a Conclusion The conclusion of your cover letter should reiterate your interest in the position, refer the recipient to any separate documents that accompany your letter and provide additional details about your qualifications (résumé, career portfolio, etc.), and thank the recipient for consideration of you as a potential candidate. The conclusion should also politely request an interview with the recipient so that you can further explain your qualifications for the job opening.

Assembling a Career Portfolio

A **career portfolio** is a collection of materials that showcases aspects of your education, training, and work experience. These professional materials are typically contained in a binder that has tabbed dividers for easy organization of the items. Many of these materials are specifically addressed in this module. However, below is a complete listing of components commonly included in a career portfolio:

- résumé
- cover letter
- references/letters of recommendation
- high school diploma
- college diploma
- college transcripts
- externship review
- certificates or licenses
- memberships in professional organizations
- awards or honors

You should bring your career portfolio to interviews. Having these professional materials is a great marketing tool for you and provides the interviewer with insight into your various qualifications for the job opening.

Completing an Online Job Application

Most companies or facilities post their job openings online. These job openings may appear on the companies' websites or may be posted on third-party websites, such as Indeed or Monster. Often, a posting on a third-party website has a link to redirect you to the company's website. If you are applying for a position on a company website, you may be directed to create a company user profile, which includes a username and a password. You would then be able to complete the company's job application. You may also need to upload and attach your résumé and, possibly, a cover letter during the application process.

Preparing for a Job Interview

Securing a desired pharmacy technician position often hinges on how well you present yourself during a job interview. For that reason, you need to devote time to interview preparation. There are seven steps to a successful interview:

1. Research the facility before your interview.
2. Confirm the type of scheduled interview.
3. Anticipate types of interview questions.
4. Practice your interviewing skills.
5. Know the location of the interview.
6. Gather your interview materials.
7. Dress to impress.

These steps are discussed in-depth in the next several pages.

> **"You need to devote time to interview preparation."**

Think It Through: Interviewing Acumen

How would you describe your interviewing skills? At what part of the interview process do you excel? What part of the interview process is a challenge for you?

Research the Facility Before Your Interview Just as the hiring manager or pharmacist-in-charge has reviewed your social media accounts before your interview, you need to do your homework as well. Before going to an interview, research the facility, including its staff and operations. You should also investigate information about the facility's culture, if possible. This information is relevant to a job seeker for two reasons: (1) It helps you determine whether the job would be a good fit for you and your skill sets, and (2) it helps you identify yourself as someone who could contribute to that culture.

To research the hiring facility, review the company's website, its profile on social networking sites, and its anonymous employee reviews on online databases. You may also want to check with other students, your externship colleagues, or acquaintances who work in a pharmacy workplace. These various sources of information are discussed below.

Hiring Facility's Website A hiring facility's website can provide you with a treasure trove of information about the company, such as the following:

- How long has the pharmacy or hospital been in business?
- Who founded the pharmacy or hospital?
- If the pharmacy is part of a chain or healthcare system, how many locations does it have?
- How many employees work at the facility? What is the management structure?

- How many current job openings exist at the pharmacy?
- What benefits does the facility offer to employees?
- What partnerships or alliances does the pharmacy have with other organizations?

You may also discover that the hiring company's website provides a description of the working culture, operations, specialty services, and any pharmacy education assistance programs the facility offers. Consider this information before you interview with the pharmacy.

Hiring Facility's Social Networking Profiles Check out the hiring facility's social networking profiles on LinkedIn, Facebook, and Twitter. A LinkedIn profile reveals information about the current employees, including their skills and backgrounds. If you are a member of LinkedIn, the facility's profile may also reveal any connections you have with the facility's current pharmacy employees. Facebook and Twitter profiles provide insights into the facility's current projects, community events, partnerships, product information, and customer feedback posts.

Online Databases of Employee Reviews Research company review websites, such as Glassdoor (**https://SSPharm.ParadigmEducation.com/Glassdoor**) or Salary (**https://SSPharm.ParadigmEducation.com/Salary**). Read the reviews but keep in mind that some of these reviews might have been posted by disgruntled employees. These reviews may be significant, however, if you see a common thread. If you detect a pattern about a specific aspect of the facility, consider this information and formulate a question for your upcoming interview based on your observations.

Communications with Others Connect with friends, externship colleagues, or others who can provide you with knowledge about the hiring facility. Consider any advice they may have about the facility before your interview.

Confirm the Type of Scheduled Interview To properly prepare for your interview, you need to know the type of interview that has been scheduled. These interview types include an online interview, a phone-screening interview, a webinar or video chat interview, a group interview, a panel interview, or a one-on-one interview.

Online Interview In this type of interview, you are provided with a series of questions to answer online. When you complete this task, you are asked to submit your responses. An online interview is sometimes timed, so be sure to read the interview instructions before you get started. Regardless of whether the interview is timed, check your responses to ensure that you have answered each question appropriately and thoroughly.

Practice Tip

If you are looking at a company's Facebook profile, make sure to click on "Visitor Posts." These postings do not show up in the main feed and can offer insight into others' experiences with the facility.

Lastly, proofread your responses for writing conventions, such as correct spelling, punctuation, capitalization, and grammar, before submitting your responses.

Note that a new online interview method has emerged that employs a similar process to the one outlined above. In this method, you may be asked to use your computer's webcam to record your responses to the interview questions rather than type them in the form fields. Your responses may be timed and, therefore, you have one opportunity to respond to each question. Because you are using a webcam, you must be dressed in professional attire, as you would for an in-person interview.

Some online interviews also include an assessment of your pharmacy math skills or critical-thinking skills. For either of these scenarios, you will be provided with instructions before the start of the interview.

Phone-Screening Interview A phone-screening interview is becoming a more common method used by hiring facilities. This initial interview process is typically conducted by a recruiter, human resources manager, or team leader. The purpose of this type of interview is for the interviewer to find out more about you and your qualifications. Based on your conversation, the interviewer will determine whether you move on to the next phase of the hiring process, which is typically an in-person interview.

Webinar/Video Chat Interview A webinar/video chat interview is set up by a hiring manager, recruiter, or team leader to allow an online video conference. Like an in-person interview, you will see and hear the representative of the hiring facility, and that representative will see and hear you. For that reason, wear appropriate professional attire and ensure that your surrounding environment is private, clean, and free of clutter. Creating a positive first impression with the hiring representative is critical to moving on in the interview process.

Group Interview In a group interview, you and other candidates for a position will be questioned in the same room at a hiring facility. Typically, all candidates are asked to respond to the same questions or statements within a designated period. Consequently, you will need to provide a focused response to each question or statement, and that response should highlight key points you wish to make. Don't get mired in too many details in your initial response. If the interviewer asks you any follow-up questions, use that time to provide additional details. The key to having a successful group interview is to provide responses that separate you from the other candidates and that provide insight into your character and skill sets.

Panel Interview In this type of interview, you will appear before a panel of multiple interviewers to respond to their questions. Typically, the panelists will provide their names and titles at the start of the interview, and

Practice Tip

If an interviewer asks for a volunteer to offer the first response to a question posed during a group interview, speak up! Volunteering to go first shows leadership, initiative, and confidence. These traits are valuable assets to a prospective employer.

then the panelists will take turns posing questions to you. During each response, you will want to maintain eye contact with the panelist asking the question but also shift your focus to the wider group at times. Respond to each question as thoroughly and thoughtfully as possible.

One-on-One Interview A one-on-one interview is a traditional type of interview in which you are interviewed by a recruiter, human resources manager, or team leader at a hiring company or facility. Be prepared, however, to have one other person join the interview at some point. A one-on-one interview provides an opportunity for you to reveal your personal qualities and interests, highlight your skill sets, and prove that you are a good fit for the position. If this interview goes well, you will be asked to return for subsequent interviews.

Anticipate Types of Interview Questions To prepare for a job interview, you need to anticipate the types of questions you might be asked. That way, you can practice your responses ahead of time. These questions typically fall into four categories: *facts*, *actions/performance*, *feelings/opinions*, or *behavioral*.

Facts Questions Facts questions cover basic information that the interviewer wants to know about you. Below are three examples of fact-based questions:

> "To prepare for a job interview, you need to anticipate the types of questions you might be asked."

- *Please tell us about yourself.* This question often sets the stage for the entire interview. You will want to briefly discuss your personal life. For example, you may want to discuss the catalyst for your interest in health care, or you may want to mention a few of your interests, such as a recreational activity or a volunteer organization. However, focus the majority of your responses on your education, work experience, and work ethic.

- *What are your salary expectations?* By asking this question, the interviewer is determining whether the salary range for the job opening aligns with your salary expectations. Do your homework before the interview by researching the salary range for entry-level pharmacy technicians in your state. You may want to ask the interviewer for the salary range of the position and reiterate that you are confident that your recent degree and certification will be rewarded in the starting salary. You may also want to provide information about your current or most recent job compensation and indicate to the interviewer that you are confident that the increased responsibilities of the job opening would be fairly compensated.

- *Describe your externship program.* This question asks for a fact-based overview of your externship experience and allows the interviewer to see the types of authentic pharmacy experiences that you have had.

Actions/Performance Questions Actions/performance questions address how you perform in a position, how you work with others, or how you achieve results. Below are three examples of actions/performance questions:

- *What are your strengths in the workplace?* This question requires you to recount workplace situations in which you have demonstrated your skills. For example, you might mention that your pharmacy preceptor noted your "excellent problem-solving ability" in your externship review. Recount for the interviewer the specific incidents that occurred in which you demonstrated that skill.

- *What are your weaknesses in the workplace?* This question can be tricky to answer well. You will want to select personal traits that can also be seen by employers as both weaknesses and strengths, depending on the circumstances. For example, you may respond, "I tend to be a perfectionist. This quality certainly lends itself to accuracy in medication dispensing. However, it also may affect the number of prescriptions that I fill." Or you may comment, "I don't have as much experience in nonsterile compounding as I would like. However, I am eager to grow in that area at your pharmacy."

- *How have you handled angry customers or colleagues in the workplace?* In this question, the interviewer wants to discern whether you have the professionalism skills to handle emotionally charged or challenging situations. As a pharmacy technician in a community or institutional pharmacy, you may be faced with difficult customers, colleagues, or providers in your daily interactions. For that reason, select a specific example from your current or past job experiences, including your externship.

Practice Tip

When responding to questions about your strengths and weaknesses, express confidence in your abilities and acknowledge your areas for growth. Understanding where you are strong and weak is an awareness that demonstrates maturity and professionalism.

Feelings/Opinions Questions Feelings/opinions questions focus on whether you will be a good fit for a company. Below are three examples of feelings/opinions questions:

- *Why are you the best candidate for this position?* This question requires a confident response. Emphasize the qualities you possess that align with the company's culture.

- *Why are you interested in this position?* This question is your chance to show the interviewer that you have done your homework! Use your response to gain a competitive edge on other job applicants by discussing the company motto or mission statement and its alignment with your personal values or attributes. For example, you might say, "In researching your company, I found that your mission statement indicates that, you value dignity and respect for both your employees and patients. The reason I chose to become a pharmacy technician is my desire to help patients. This desire comes from the great respect I had for my grandparents, whom I helped with their medication therapy. Therefore, I feel that I would be a great candidate for this position."

- *Describe your ideal supervisor.* This question allows the interviewer to determine how well you would fit with the working style of the supervisor who will oversee the job opening. Answer honestly and provide reasons why this type of supervisor would mesh with your personality, work ethic, and career goals.

Behavioral Questions Behavioral questions focus on the job applicant's ability to solve problems, collaborate with others, and handle conflict. Often the introduction to behavioral questions is as follows: "Tell me about a time when. . . ." These questions provide an interviewer with insight into your overall skills and competencies. The challenge with these types of questions is that they require detailed, multifaceted answers. If these answers are not crafted beforehand, it can be easy to get off track and end up not answering the questions well.

> "Behavioral questions provide an interviewer with insight into your overall skills . . . ."

The best way to craft a response for most behavioral questions is to structure your response using the S.T.A.R. method:

Situation: Describe the situation in the example you are providing, such as the workplace setting where it occurred, your position at that workplace, etc.

Task: Explain the action or objective that was assigned or necessary for completion.

Approach: Discuss the approach or strategy that you used to achieve the task.

Results: Describe the outcome of the situation, objective, or task.

Below are three examples of behavioral questions:

- *Describe a time when you recognized a problem and took the initiative to address it.* This question requires a detailed response, such as the following:

I was an extern at MyTown Hospital. While on the floor, I noticed that the Pyxis machines in many of the med rooms showed wear and tear and that the screens were smudged due to constant use *(Situation)*. I asked my preceptor if, during downtime, I could clean the machines while not in use *(Task)*. I was assigned one hour during each of my shifts to clean them. I took microfiber cloths and cleaning solution and wiped down the machines and keyboards, as well as the screens and biometric scanners *(Approach)*. The nursing staff was very surprised and thankful for my efforts, and my preceptor nominated me for a service excellence award for going above and beyond in my work *(Results)*.

- *Tell me about a time when you skillfully managed a conflict while working as a member of a team.* This question requires a detailed response, such as the following:

  While I was an employee at a retail store, I worked with an employee who enjoyed gossiping about our manager (Situation). I did not want to add to a toxic work environment, but I also did not want to upset my coworker, whom I had to work with on a constant basis, and I had to figure out a way to manage both outcomes in a positive manner *(Task)*. During a work break, I approached my co-worker and explained that I valued our friendship but was not interested in engaging in gossip about our manager, as it made me uncomfortable *(Approach)*. The coworker understood my position and respected my wishes. Because there was not another coworker to gossip with on our shift, my coworker promptly stopped *(Results)*.

- *Describe a time when you handled a difficult customer effectively.* This question is commonly asked during a hiring interview for a community pharmacy technician and requires a detailed response, such as the following:

  I completed my externship at MyTown Community Pharmacy and was working at the prescription intake window *(Situation)*. A customer came to the window and was agitated that none of the five pharmacies, including this pharmacy, would fill a Norco prescription *(Task)*. I proceeded to ask the customer for the names of the pharmacies that would not fill the prescription. I explained that the policy at this pharmacy was to fill a Norco prescription only for new patients with a cancer diagnosis. I went on to explain that the pharmacy was allotted a limited monthly amount of Norco for our existing customers. I also offered the names of other facilities that may have different policies and a larger allotment of the medication *(Approach)*. Because I explained the process and reasoning rather than just saying "No, we can't help you," the customer was more understanding and thanked me for the advice *(Results)*.

Practice Your Interviewing Skills Your job-search preparation should include sharpening your interview skills. To practice your skills, participate in a mock interview. A mock interview is a role-playing activity in which one individual assumes the role of an interviewee (in this case, you) and one individual assumes the role of an interviewer. Conducting a mock interview helps you rehearse answers to common interview questions, think on your feet when asked unexpected questions, construct logical and coherent responses, and improve the way you present yourself.

To set up a mock interview, ask a family member or friend to be the interviewer and explain the purpose of the activity: to provide you with honest feedback on your interviewing skills. If the individual agrees to participate, arrange for a meeting time and supply the individual with a list of common interview questions to ask you. Encourage the interviewer to add a few unexpected questions to this list. These questions often present a what-would-you-do scenario and ask the interviewee to explain a course of action to address the situation. For example, an unexpected question that a pharmacy technician candidate might need to address is, "What would you do if you witnessed one of your colleagues diverting drugs?" Explain to the interviewer that asking an unexpected question is a common practice in a hiring interview because companies value employees who think quickly on their feet and demonstrate problem-solving skills.

As the interviewee, research the company before participating in the mock interview, just as you would for a real job interview. Choose a pharmacy for your interviewer to represent during the interview; then spend time learning about the facility and its operations. This research serves two purposes in an interview: You can convey knowledge about the pharmacy during questioning, and you can prepare questions for the interviewer about the hiring facility. Asking questions of an interviewer shows that you are interested in learning more about the company. (For detailed information on asking questions during an interview, see the section titled "Posing Questions to the Interviewer" later in this module.)

Before the mock interview, recreate a typical one-on-one interview setting and don appropriate professional attire. Establish a period for the interview (e.g., 30 minutes), and set a timer to remind you. You may also want to consider recording the interview so that you can critique your responses; observe your posture, nonverbal communication, and eye contact; and listen to the tone, pace, and volume of your voice.

After the mock interview, ask for feedback from the interviewer on your performance. Note the areas in which you did well and the areas in which you need to improve. Continue to hone your interview skills in preparation for your job search.

Know the Location of Your Interview Once you have secured a hiring interview, familiarize yourself with the location of the facility where the interview will be conducted. To do so, conduct a trial run by mapping out the route to the facility and driving yourself or taking public transportation to reach your destination. Time yourself so that you have a baseline for how long it takes to get to the facility. Then be sure to add additional time for traffic concerns, which is especially important if your interview is scheduled when rush-hour traffic is peaking. You should also allow time for road construction or alternate routes that you may need to take.

Practice Tip

Plan to arrive for a job interview at least 15 to 30 minutes early, and make sure that you know the name of your contact person at the facility.

Gather Your Interview Materials Before your interview, gather materials that you will need for your meeting:

- a blue or black pen
- a notebook for taking notes
- a few copies of your cover letter
- a few copies of your résumé printed on high-quality paper
- your career portfolio containing copies of letters of recommendation, honors and awards, and education transcripts

Be sure to organize these items for easy access during the interview.

Dress to Impress Various studies have revealed that hiring managers often make a preliminary decision about a job candidate within 90 seconds after meeting that individual. For that reason, you need to create a strong first impression before you even begin the interview process. First impressions can be created by several factors, such as friendliness, eye contact, or a handshake. However, your professional appearance weighs heavily in how you are judged by others.

Regardless of your personal style or taste, you should adapt your image to the acceptable dress code or standards of the hiring company or facility (see the Workplace Wisdom feature box below). An unwillingness to conform is a choice. Making the choice to avoid conformity for an interview or for a job may mean that you are limiting your options in finding employment.

Practice Tip

Remember to always dress up for a job interview. Many qualified individuals have lost out on a job because they were underdressed for an interview.

WORKPLACE WISDOM

Professional Appearance Guidelines
Below are several guidelines to follow when projecting a professional appearance at a job interview.

Hygiene
- Shower or bathe before your interview.
- Brush your teeth.
- Make sure that your fingernails are clean.
- Avoid wearing perfume or cologne.

Hair and Makeup
- Shampoo and comb your hair before your interview.
- Trim or remove facial or body hair as necessary.
- Apply natural-looking makeup, if you wear any.

Clothing
- Make sure that your interview clothes are clean and pressed.
- Wear attire that is conservative in color and fit.
- Choose clothing options that cover body tattoos.
- Avoid hats or head coverings unless they are worn for cultural or religious reasons.

Shoes
- Wear professional footwear.
- Be sure that your shoes are clean and well-polished.

Jewelry
- Remove facial piercings.
- Wear conservative jewelry.

Therefore, be sure to dress in professional attire and employ good hygiene practices. For more detailed information on professional appearance, refer to Module 3.

9.4 Job Interview Success

Now that you have invested time in preparing for a job interview, focus on conducting a successful job interview. Be sure that you arrive a few minutes early and have the necessary materials in hand. Tell the receptionist the name of your contact person (either a recruiter, human resources manager, or team leader) as well as your name so that your contact person can be informed that you have arrived.

> ### Think It Through: Impressions Matter
> Pretend that you are a pharmacist-in-charge about to meet a potential candidate for a pharmacy technician position at your pharmacy. What aspects about the candidate's appearance or behavior would make a good impression? What aspects would make a bad impression?

Making a Good First Impression

Work Wise

In his book *Blink: The Power of Thinking without Thinking*, Malcolm Gladwell states that individuals make choices, such as first impressions, in the blink of an eye. In fact, Gladwell asserts that first impressions occur in as little as 15 seconds!

As mentioned earlier, a first impression is critical. Greet your interviewer with a smile and a firm handshake. Be personable by engaging in light conversation before the interview. Once your interview begins, the interviewer will be observing your **demeanor**, or your outward behavior manifested by your nonverbal communication, attitude, manners, and personality. (For detailed information on nonverbal communication, refer to Module 5.) The interviewer will also be assessing your degree of **articulation**, or the ability to speak and express yourself effectively.

Staying Focused in Your Responses

Your interview preparation will help you stay focused and avoid a major pitfall during the interview process: **rambling**. Often a sign of anxiety or nervousness, rambling is an aimless or unfocused discussion that goes in many directions and is hard for a listener to follow. To avoid rambling, address each interview question by providing the appropriate amount of information (detailed, but not too detailed) in the appropriate amount of time.

Two strategies you can use when responding to a question is to pause before you respond and follow an established format in your responses. The format to your response has three parts: (1) Provide a one-sentence statement that addresses the question directly; (2) add details to your response by presenting facts or experiences that support your one-sentence statement; and (3) offer a final concluding statement that summarizes your response. Note how a three-pronged approach works with this sample interview question:

Interview Question: What was the most rewarding experience you had in your last position?

During my externship at a hospital pharmacy, I caught a medication error that could have had serious consequences for patients *(One-Sentence Statement)*. I was filling an out-of-stock report for the Pyxis machine and noticed that the medication I was pulling looked different from what it typically does. The medication on the shelf was supposed to be methylprednisolone sodium succinate (Solu-Medrol). It was, in fact, methylprednisolone acetate (Depo-Medrol). This discrepancy was the result of a restocking error *(Details)*. Because I asked my supervisor about the medication, I prevented a serious medication error *(Concluding Statement)*.

Demonstrating Honesty in Your Interview

When responding to each question, be sure that you provide honest answers. Don't use **hyperbole**, or exaggerated statements or claims about your experience or skill sets. If you don't have a particular experience or skill set, be truthful with the interviewer. Indicate your willingness to learn that task or skill according to the procedures outlined by the hiring facility. Explain to the interviewer that having no prior experience in a specific process could be perceived as a benefit because you have no preconceived notions about how the process is performed in other facilities.

Posing Questions to the Interviewer

A typical job interview ends with the interviewer asking if you have any questions. Take advantage of this opportunity by posing questions and then taking notes when you receive the answers. Asking questions at the close of an interview shows that you have prepared well for the interview, have listened intently during the interview, and are interested in being considered for the position. Below are some possible lines of questioning:

- *Ask a follow-up question to something you learned during the interview.* For example, a follow-up question to learning about the roles and responsibilities of a pharmacy technician in this facility might be, "What are the specific tasks of a pharmacy technician in the medication reconciliation process in your facility?"

- *Inquire about something you discovered in your company research.* For example, a follow-up question might be, "I see that your pharmacy has a partnership with the United Nations Foundation. Social responsibility is important to me. Can you tell me more about that partnership?"

Work Wise

Honesty is an important trait for a pharmacy employee. As a pharmacist with many years of experience once said, "I can train a technician how to do almost anything. I cannot untrain dishonesty."

- *Inquire about a recent news item regarding the positive actions of the company or facility.* For example, a follow-up question might be, "I read in the newspaper that your facility recently installed a drug disposal machine. Could you tell me about the background and purpose of that initiative?"

Leaving a Good Last Impression

Just as creating a good first impression is critical in a job interview, so too is leaving a good last impression. To leave a good last impression with the interviewer, be sure that you address these final items:

- *Ask about next steps in the hiring process.* Clarify the time frame for the hiring process and ask how and when you will be informed about your candidacy for the position. If you have not received any feedback within that time frame, contact the interviewer for a status update.
- *Make any necessary notes about the job interview or the hiring facility shortly after the interview.* Review these notes to create follow-up questions for a subsequent interview at this facility or to help you weigh the pros and cons of different positions after participating in interviews for several companies.
- *Send a follow-up email to the interviewer.* Within 24 hours of the interview, send an email to the interviewer. The email should express your gratitude for the opportunity to interview with the company or facility; your confidence that the position would be a good fit for your personality, education, training and skill sets; and your hopefulness that you will receive positive news about your candidacy.

9.5 Career Management

Practice Tip

Goal setting is a continual process, not a one-time event. Review your goals periodically to determine whether they still align with your priorities and are still achievable.

Although securing an entry-level position is your first priority when you are finished with your postsecondary education, you should also look ahead to career management. Managing your professional career involves understanding the goal-setting process, building SMART goals, establishing short-term and long-term career goals, creating your own Career Success Plan, and networking.

Setting Your Goals

As you begin your career as a pharmacy technician, you need to have a good understanding of goal setting so that you can work toward personal and professional career goals. Goal setting also has an empowering effect: You are in charge of your own career journey and end destination.

Knowing how to set a goal is a skill that does not come naturally for most individuals. The process must be learned, and it begins with self-reflection and introspection. Consider the following criteria when setting a professional goal:

- *The goal must be your own.* A goal that is dictated by someone else is difficult to accomplish and rarely achieved. You should be the person deciding your goals.
- *The goal must be challenging yet attainable.* Setting a realistic, achievable goal provides you with the incentive to stay focused and maintain a positive attitude while making progress toward achieving that goal.
- *The goal must be inspired and fit your value*s. Having an ideal to aspire to or an admired person to emulate can help you set and achieve a goal.
- *The goal must have benefits you can picture.* Having a vision of your goal and knowing the benefits associated with its achievement can help you persevere when you are facing obstacles.

To gauge your ability to set goals, refer to the Self-Reflection feature below.

Self-Reflection:
How Would You Gauge Your Goal-Setting Ability?

For each of the statements, mark the appropriate box to rate your goal-setting ability: "always," "sometimes," or "rarely/never." Respond to statements as honestly as possible.

Statement	Always	Sometimes	Rarely/Never
I set goals with specific descriptions that measure their success.			
I describe the personal rewards of reaching my goals.			
I choose goals that are challenging but achievable.			
I visualize my goal-setting process and picture myself achieving these goals.			
I consider potential obstacles and how to avoid or overcome them.			
I give myself deadlines, so I won't procrastinate.			
I identify subgoals or tasks required to achieve the primary goal.			
I accurately estimate the time it takes to achieve the goals.			
I regularly monitor my progress toward completing the goals.			
I adapt my goals as necessary to fit circumstances.			
Subtotal per column	____ x5	____ x3	____ x 1

Tally Your Score: Always = 5 points; Sometimes = 3 points; Rarely/Never = 1 point

Total Score: _____

Continues…

31 to 50 points: This score indicates that you have a strong foundation in goal setting. Use the goal-setting techniques described in this module to help you refine those skills.

11 to 30 points: This score indicates that you have some familiarity and success with goal setting. However, use the goal-setting techniques

described in this module to achieve your unmet goals and improve your success rate.

Below 11 points: This score indicates that you are not using goal-setting techniques. Establish a plan as to how to implement the goal-setting techniques described in this module in all tasks.

Establish Long-Term and Short-Term Career Goals To begin your own career planning, set a **long-term career goal**. This goal is your end goal or destination of your career journey and typically requires three to five years to achieve. The steps you take to reach your long-term career goal are considered **short-term career goals**. These goals are the stopping points along your journey and typically require one to three years to achieve.

For example, perhaps your long-term career goal is to become a sterile compounding technician. This pharmacy position is typically not an entry-level position for a pharmacy technician. To reach this advanced role, you will need work experience and additional training and education in that specific area of pharmacy practice. Often, individuals pursuing the end goal of becoming sterile compounding technicians begin their careers in community pharmacies and then move into hospital or institutional pharmacies. Once in hospital or institutional settings, they undergo specialized training in sterile compounding and aseptic technique. Finally, they sit for the CSPT exam. Consequently, these actions or steps that pharmacy technicians take to achieve their long-term career goal are considered short-term goals or objectives.

EXPAND YOUR KNOWLEDGE

Advanced Roles for Pharmacy Technicians

When setting a long-term career goal, consider several advanced roles that pharmacy technicians can assume after work experience, specialized training, and/or additional certification. Examples of these advanced roles include the following:

- automation specialist
- compliance officer
- controlled substance technician
- diabetes education technician

- inventory management technician
- investigational drug technician
- lead technician
- medication reconciliation technician
- patient assistance technician
- pharmacy technician marketer
- pharmacy technician supervisor
- sterile compounding technician
- tech-check-tech

Build SMART Goals To ensure that your long-term and short-term career goals are constructive and realistic, follow the criteria outlined in the acronym *SMART*:

- *Specific:* Long-term and short-term career goals need to be specific or detailed. For example, you might express the following long-term career goal to your pharmacy supervisor during a performance review: "My long-term career goal is to find a position as a medication reconciliation technician in the emergency department of this hospital."

- *Measurable:* Long-term and short-term career goals need to be measurable so that there is evidence of accomplishment. For example, a measurable short-term career goal toward securing your desired long-term goal of being a medication reconciliation technician might be the following: "One of my short-term career goals is to pass a competency exam for medication reconciliation that my hospital offers to pharmacy technicians."

- *Achievable:* Long-term and short-term career goals need to be achievable. For example, an attainable short-term career goal for becoming a medication reconciliation technician might be the following: "A short-term career goal I have is to be trained on my hospital's template documentation system, known as a T-System, so that I can document a patient's medication history accurately."

- *Relevant:* Long-term and short-term career goals must be relevant to the time, place, role, and desired outcomes. For example, you may want to set the following short-term career goal: "One of my short-term career goals is to complete a patient's medication history before admission orders and to track my progress to meet that goal."

- *Time-bound:* Long-term and short-term career goals must have deadlines to avoid procrastination. Deadlines measure incremental progress that leads to the completion of short-term career goals and, consequently, to the fulfillment of a long-term career goal. For example, you may want to set the following long-term career goal: "My long-term career goal is to become a medication reconciliation technician within three years."

Creating a Career Success Plan

Now that you understand the importance of goal setting in your professional career, you are ready to consider your own goals and the actions to take to achieve those goals. Creating a Career Success Plan will help you assemble and organize your ideas. The following components should be included in a Career Success Plan:

- Long-term career goal and a time frame for its completion
- Short-term career goals and a time frame for the completion of each goal
- Actions and criteria to gauge the success of your short-term career goals
- Resources to keep you focused and moving forward
- Individuals or mentors who can guide you or support you in your career journey

To help you formulate your own Career Success Plan, refer to Table 9.2. This Career Success Plan was created by Jamilla, a recent college graduate of a pharmacy technician program.

Table 9.2 Jamilla's Career Success Plan

Long-Term Career Goal: To become a senior pharmacy technician in five years

Short-Term Career Goals	Actions to Achieve Short-Term Career Goals	Success Criteria	Due Date	Resources Needed	Helpful Individuals or Mentors
Complete pharmacy technician certification exam	• Research test certification standards and use online resource materials to prepare for exam • Save money for required exam fee • Apply for and schedule date to sit for the exam	Attain CPhT	End of current calendar year	• Exam preparation materials • Exam fee • Transportation to testing center	Professor Mizuki Kakisoko in my pharmacy technician program at school
Accept a pharmacy technician position in a hospital pharmacy	Apply for available pharmacy technician positions at hospital pharmacies	Secure a pharmacy technician position at Pelican Lake Medical Center	One to two years after graduation from training program	Career portfolio, including résumé, cover letter, references, college transcripts, certification, and awards	My sister, a registered nurse at Pelican Lake Medical Center

Continues...

Short-Term Career Goals	Actions to Achieve Short-Term Career Goals	Success Criteria	Due Date	Resources Needed	Helpful Individuals or Mentors
Receive a promotion to a senior pharmacy technician position at Pelican Lake Medical Center	• Receive excellent annual job performance reviews • Work collaboratively with other healthcare team members • Complete additional didactic training in the prevention, identification, and reporting of medication errors • Complete an advanced pharmacy calculations course • Perform filling evaluations with 100% accuracy	• Receive a positive recommendation for a promotion • Accept the senior pharmacy technician position and earn a higher salary	Three to five years after entry-level pharmacy technician position	• Career portfolio, including résumé, cover letter, references, college transcripts, certification, and awards • Completion of prerequisite didactic training as required by the medical center	Dr. Bertoli, director of pharmacy

9.6 Module Summary

Now that you are making the transition from the academic setting to the professional workplace, you should be aware of the career competencies that employers are looking for in their employees. One of these areas is career management.

Launching a career requires self-awareness and planning. The first step is achieving pharmacy technician national certification, which conveys to an employer a higher level of commitment and competency as a pharmacy technician. To prepare for a pharmacy technician certification exam—either the PTCE (offered by the PTCB) or the ExCPT (offered by the NHA)—seek information on the organization's website. Be aware that you will be required to take continuing education credits for certification renewal.

Career preparation also requires researching information on career options and exploring avenues for entering the job market, such as career fairs and recruiting companies. You will also want to review your social media accounts and prepare your career portfolio, which includes your résumé, cover letter, references, transcripts, externship review, certificates/licenses, and awards/honors.

Practice Tip

Make sure that you review your progress on a weekly or monthly basis. Celebrate the small achievements toward reaching your short-term and long-term career goals. This review will help you to keep moving forward.

Preparing for your job interview is the final step in your job search. That preparation might involve researching the facility, confirming the type of interview, anticipating the types of questions, and practicing your interviewing skills.

Finally, you will want to consider your career trajectory by setting constructive and realistic short-term and long-term goals. Creating a Career Success Plan can help you organize your goals, establish actions and success criteria for each goal, and set realistic time frames in which to meet each goal. With the ever-expanding roles of pharmacy technicians, you have the opportunity to advance into many specific areas of pharmacy, such as investigational drugs, medication reconciliation, and sterile compounding.

 The online course includes additional review and assessment resources.

Career Readiness & Externships: Soft Skills for Pharmacy Technicians

Index

Image Credits

Page 46, © Shutterstock.com/Dragon Images; *page 47*, © Shutterstock.com/Rob Marmion; *page 51*,
© Shutterstock.com/Syda Productions; *page 54*, © Shutterstock.com/Andrii Zastrozhnov; *page 57*, (both)
© Shutterstock.com/Lemurik; *page 58*, (both) © Shutterstock.com/stockfour; *page 78*, © Dreamstime.com/
Czaroot.

Appendix A

ASHP/ACPE Accreditation Standards

The following identifies the *ASHP/ACPE Accreditation Standards* addressed in each module of Paradigm's *Career Readiness & Externships: Soft Skills for Pharmacy Technicians*. This appendix identifies the *ASHP/ACPE Standards* associated with the module content. This list is meant for guidance purposes only and was created by the author of this text. Neither ASHP nor ACPE has participated in or had any role in creating the list of standards or any other content that is included in this book.

Module 1. Time Management
   Entry-Level: 1.6

Module 2. Critical Thinking & Problem Solving
   Entry-Level: 1.8
   Advanced-Level: 1.10

Module 3. Professional Appearance
   Entry-Level: 1.2

Module 4. Professional Behavior
   Entry-Level: 1.2
   Advanced-Level: 1.12

Module 5. Professional Communications
   Entry-Level: 1.3, 1.4, 1.7
   Advanced-Level: 1.12

Module 6. Multicultural Awareness & Cultural Competency
   Entry-Level: 1.5
   Advanced-Level: 1.12

Module 7. Law & Ethics
   Entry-Level: 1.1, 5.1 to 5.5
   Advanced-Level: 5.9

Module 8. Externship Preparation & Practice
   Entry-Level: 1.2, 1.5, 1.6, 1.7
   Advanced-Level: 1.10

Module 9. Career Readiness, Planning, & Management
   Entry-Level: 1.2, 1.4, 1.6, 1.7, 2.1